PARAMEDIC EMERGENCY CARE EXAM REVIEW

second edition

Keyed to Paramedic Emergency Care 3E

RICHARD A. CHERRY

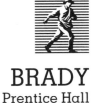

BRADY
Prentice Hall
Upper Saddle River, New Jersey 07458

Publisher: Susan Katz
Editorial Assistant: Carol Sobel
Director of Production and Manufacturing:
    Bruce Johnson
Manufacturing Buyer: Ilene Sanford

Managing Production Editor: Patrick Walsh
Production Editor: Robin Lucas
Printer/Binder: Banta Harrisonburg
Cover Design: Miguel Ortiz

Printed in the United State of America
10 9 8 7 6 5 4

ISBN 0-8359-5103-0

PRENTICE-HALL INTERNATIONAL (UK) LIMITED, *London*
PRENTICE-HALL OF AUSTRALIA PTY. LIMITED, *Sydney*
PRENTICE-HALL CANADA INC., *Toronto*
PRENTICE-HALL HISPANOAMERICANA, S.A., *MEXICO*
PRENTICE-HALL OF INDIA PRIVATE LIMITED, *New Delhi*
PRENTICE-HALL OF JAPAN, INC., *Tokyo*
SIMON & SCHUSTER ASIA PTE. LTD., *Singapore*
EDITORA PRENTICE-HALL DO BRASIL, LTDA., *Rio de Janeiro*

To Dr. Mike Jastremski, who believed in me when no one else did.

Contents

To the Student

The future belongs to those who believe in the beauty of their dreams.

Eleanor Roosevelt

This book is designed to help you prepare for both your certification exams and for the streets. I have provided for you over 1,000 multiple choice questions covering every chapter of *Paramedic Emergency Care* (PEC) and the USDOT Paramedic Curriculum. The questions test your knowledge, your understanding, and your ability to apply your knowledge in emergency medical scenarios. These scenarios are designed to help you develop the judgment necessary to solve real medical problems of real people. I also have provided the correct answer to each question, the rationale for the answer, and the page number from *Paramedic Emergency Care* where you will find more detailed explanation. The final ingredient is desire, which you must provide.

The great American poet, Henry David Thoreau once wrote, "If one advances confidently in the direction of his dreams and endeavors to live the life which he has imagined, he will meet with a success unexpected in common hours." *Kaizen* is a Japanese word that means making a lifelong commitment toward self-improvement. This Oriental philosophy encourages life satisfaction through continual personal and professional growth. It is a neverending process of making small, incremental improvements in your life. If there was ever a group of people who should adopt the Kaizen philosophy in their lives, it's EMS providers. Turning your professional life into an endless quest for perfection brings with it a measure of success. It is the journey—not the goal—that enriches our lives. It's like taking a cruise. The object is not to get to your destination as quickly as possible but to have fun getting there. Likewise, success is not a destination, but a journey. When you make this commitment, you begin to reap the rewards immediately. The moment you set sail on this course, you and your future patients benefit from your increased commitment. Providing emergency medical care is a tremendous privilege. With this privilege comes responsibility to do your very best academic work. Think about how much patient care you will affect. Think about how many people's lives you will influence. Do so and you should begin to realize the tremendous responsibility you accept when you bear the title of "paramedic."

The formula is simple. Turn your weaknesses into your strengths. The first step is to identify your weak areas. This step is difficult, but critical. It's not easy because you must admit that you're not doing the job you could be doing. It's much easier to become complacent about your abilities. It's much easier to become comfortable with your present performance and accept your limitations as such. The consequences of this kind of attitude, however, are alarming. Patients suffer from your lack of knowledge and skill. Use this book of questions to identify your weak areas.

Once you have identified your weaknesses make the personal commitment to improve in those areas. World-class athletes measure improvements by fractions of seconds and inches. They work tirelessly on making tiny improvements in the many aspects of their sport. They call it "personal best." You can achieve your personal best each year by making small incremental improvements in the needed areas. By improving just one aspect of your craft each year, you make great strides. The short-term results are immediate—you enjoy EMS more because you are becoming better at it. We all enjoy doing the things that we do well. The long-term result is a rewarding career caring for those who are sick or injured.

Former Green Bay Packer football coach Vince Lombardi best described this attitude when he wrote, "Making the effort to be perfect is what life is all about. If you will not settle for anything less than the best, you will be amazed at what you can do with your lives. Winning isn't everything, but making the effort to win is. The difference between a successful person and an unsuccessful one is not a lack of knowledge, or a lack of strength, but a lack of will."

Remember, this is a lifelong journey. Don't try to do it all by Friday, but never give up your quest. You build a successful life one day at a time.

Someone once asked Miami Dolphin football coach Don Shula if it wasn't a waste of time trying to correct such a small flaw in his team's offense. Don's reply was "What's a small flaw?" That's striving for perfection. That's a commitment to excellence. That's Kaizen. It's no wonder that his 1972 squad is still the only team ever to complete a perfect season. It's also no wonder that he is the winningest coach in professional football history.

Why make learning a lifelong endeavor? American humorist Will Rogers once said, "Even if you are on the right track, you'll get run over if you just stand there." He was right. I don't believe in the status quo. Either you're getting better or you're getting worse. It's like walking up a down escalator. If you keep moving forward, you'll eventually end up on top. You will at least stay in place. Once you slow down or stop, however, you begin to move downwards until you eventually reach the bottom. A paramedic who fails to keep pace with the fast-moving world of emergency medicine soon becomes obsolete, even dangerous. This book is designed to help you maintain a high level of paramedic knowledge.

The road to excellence is not easy. It's easier to take the path of least resistance. It's easier to back away from excellence than it is to give everything you've got. While it's easier to let frustrations, distractions, and fatigue erode your performance, it's not satisfying in the long run. Making this commitment takes a tremendous amount of courage. If you fail, there are no excuses. You can look yourself in the mirror and know that you gave it your very best. In that effort, you have not failed. When your paramedic career is over, you want to look back with no regrets.

Do you want to be great? Many talk the talk, few walk the walk. Many want to be great, but few are willing to pay the price. What is "average?" According to Notre Dame football coach Lou Holtz, "It's the best of the worst or the worst of the best. It's the top of the bottom or the bottom of the top. It's nowhere." Challenge yourself to make a commitment to excellence. If you believe in yourself, you can be as great as you want to be. You must have the courage, the determination, the dedication, and the competitive drive to do it. You must be willing to sacrifice the little things in life and pay the price for the things that are worthwhile. If you can do all these things, great things can happen.

Once you have made a commitment to a way of life, you put the greatest strength in the world behind you. We call it "heart." Once you have made this commitment, nothing will stop you short of success. You have to want to. You have to have a raging desire to be the best you can be. It's not a part-time thing. Athletes call it "competitive anger" and many use this motivational factor to spur them onto greatness. There have been few successful people that didn't have competitive anger driving their talents to the surface. Hall of Fame baseball player Ted Williams once said, "I wanted to be the greatest hitter who ever lived. A man has to have goals—for a day, for a lifetime—and that was mine, to have people say, 'There goes Ted Williams, the greatest hitter who ever lived.'" He was the greatest hitter because he made an unwavering commitment to excellence.

To succeed, you don't have to be the most experienced or the talented, just the most tenacious. You must hold on to your goals and dreams. Your rewards for making a commitment to excellence cannot be measured financially. You will have the feeling of confidence and self-worth from having accomplished something for yourself. This feeling will transfer into other areas of your life in more ways than you can ever imagine.

The essence of Kaizen is adopting a positive attitude about everything you do. According to this philosophy, attitude is the most important thing you can develop in your life. While ability determines capability, attitude determines performance. You were born with certain abilities. Your attitude determines how close you come to realizing your full potential. Don't dwell on your shortcomings and limitations. Try to work around them. My father used to tell me that things turn out the best for those who make the best out of the way things turn out. Turn your weaknesses into strengths. Then measure yourself not by what you have done, but by what you have done with your ability.

You don't have to be a sports fan to appreciate the tremendous difference a positive attitude makes. Victory doesn't always go to the strongest or fastest but to the one who wants it more. A positive attitude means believing in miracles. In sports, there are countless stories of people who overcame overwhelming odds to achieve their personal best. These people conceived the inconceivable, and then did it. When we hear of these triumphs, our usual response is "unbelievable."

With the proper attitude, you can do great things. Penn State Football coach Joe Paterno describes this phenomenon: "The power of concentrating your brain, your whole body, your whole nervous system, your adrenaline, all your will on a single goal is an almost unbeatable concentration of force." David may have understood this before he went up against Goliath. After watching the 1980 United States Olympic Hockey team win the gold medal in Lake Placid, I know I do. Anything is possible.

A positive attitude means making the best of your abilities. Pete Rose was not born with great strength, size, or speed. His God-given talents were few. His most important talent was his attitude. No one got more out of himself on a baseball diamond than Pete Rose. As Pulitzer Prize winning sports columnist Jim Murray wrote, "God made Babe Ruth and Mickey Mantle baseball players. Pete Rose made Pete Rose one."

A competitor finds a way to win. Competitors take bad breaks and use them to drive themselves just that much harder. Quitters take bad breaks and use them as reasons to give up. It's all a matter of pride. You'll never know what you can do unless you try. Life is short. Try as hard as you can. You owe it to your future patients and, especially, to yourself.

A positive attitude means adopting the work ethic. The only place where success comes before hard work is in the dictionary. Athletics teaches the self-discipline of hard work and sacrifice necessary to reach a goal. Nowadays, too many people are looking for a shortcut. They want a free ride, a handout. For athletes this shouldn't be true because they know what it takes. There are no short cuts to success. Just the blood, sweat, and tears that produce results. Life resembles athletics. You must work hard to achieve anything. It's like the bank. Unless you make a deposit, you cannot make a withdrawal.

Some people say that good things happen to those who wait. I say that great things happen to those who work. American poet Robert Frost once wrote, "The world is full of willing people, some willing to work, others willing to let them." Boy was he right. Don't spend your professional life on the sidelines watching others achieve greatness. Do it yourself. Make the effort to work *harder* to overcome your weaknesses.

A positive attitude means never becoming complacent and satisfied with the job you do. Always try to do it better. Develop an insatiable appetite for perfection. Like the writer who writes a bestseller wants to create another one. Like the painter who creates a masterpiece wants to paint another one. Like the lawyer who wins the most prominent case in the nation wants to try another one. It doesn't mean they have to do it. The great ones want to do it again. Great paramedics never end their search for better ways to treat their patients.

What are your weaknesses? Successful dieters say the best way to get started on a diet is to stand naked in front of a mirror (without holding in your stomach) for an honest evaluation. That's what this book is all about. Be self-critical and make small improvements in those areas that need it most. Be patient. As any weekend golfer can tell you, improvement comes slowly. The difference between the possible and the impossible lies in your determination. You must have goals and dreams if you are ever going to do anything in this world. Set your goals in life, and go after them with all the drive, self-confidence, and determination that you possess.

Good luck!

Acknowledgments

There are three people I would like to thank for their help in preparing this manuscript:

Bob McCaffrey, a former paramedic student of mine, reviewed each page of this book and offered his insight as to what questions and information were most helpful. His constant battle cry, "Who cares about this?" kept me constantly focused on the practical side of paramedic street medicine. Bob was a tremendous asset to me during this project.

Wendy Ranc, my secretary, transcribed the majority of this book. But it was her help in attending to the many administrative details of our paramedic program that freed me up to finish this project. Wendy has been and, hopefully, will continue to be an outstanding resource to me.

Mike Cunningham, D.O., is a former resident in Emergency Medicine at the SUNY Health Science Center in Syracuse. A good friend of mine, Mike helped teach our paramedic students each year of his residency and was an invaluable asset to our program. Mike contributed the extra pharmacology section of this book.

DIVISION 1—
PREHOSPITAL ENVIRONMENT

CHAPTER 1

Roles and Responsibilities of the Paramedic

QUESTIONS

1. EMS prior to the late 1960's was characterized by
   A. fast, horizontal transport
   B. elaborate communications networks
   C. intensive training programs
   D. strict medical direction

2. How did Dr. J. Frank Pantridge of Belfast, Ireland plant the seed for prehospital emergency care?
   A. He trained the first paramedics
   B. He brought ALS to the patient
   C. He developed a way to send ECG by radio
   D. He authored the "White Paper"

3. The physician credited with training the first paramedics in the United States is
   A. Dr. J. Frank Pantridge
   B. Dr. Eugene Nagel
   C. Dr. Mickey Eisenberg
   D. Dr. Jeffrey Clawson

4. The rules that govern the conduct of members of a particular group or are called
   A. ethics

     B. morals

     C. standards

     D. principles

5. Professionalism is exhibited by all of the following **EXCEPT**

     A. setting high standards

     B. seeking self improvement

     C. earning the respect of your peers

     D. aiming for the minimum standard

6. Which of the following is **NOT** an on-scene duty of the paramedic?

     A. Patient care

     B. Leadership

     C. Certification

     D. Customer service

7. The process by which an agency or association grants recognition to an individual who has met its qualifications is known as

     A. licensure

     B. certification

     C. reciprocity

     D. censure

8. The process by which a governmental agency grants permission to engage in a given occupation to an individual who has attained the degree of competency required to ensure the public's protection is known as

     A. licensure

     B. certification

     C. reciprocity

     D. censure

9. The process by which an agency grants credentials to an individual who has comparable credentials from another agency is known as

     A. licensure

     B. certification

     C. reciprocity

     D. consensus

10. NASAR, NAEMSP, and NAEMT are examples of

     A. professional organizations

     B. EMS journals

     C. licensing agencies

     D. national testing agencies

11. Which of the following is **NOT** a responsibility of the National Registry?

     A. Administering testing materials

     B. Establishing national standards

     C. Assisting in evaluating training programs

     D. Licensing and certifying EMT's in each state

12. Paramedics spend the majority of their time

     A. answering emergency calls

B. in self-preparation
C. providing patient care
D. answering system-abuse calls

ANSWERS **1. ANS—A** *PEC—5*

Prior to the late 1960's, EMS was characterized by fast horizontal transport, crude rescue, and little training. There was no physician direction, communications, or specialized emergency medical knowledge. When people died, it was "meant to be". The public did not expect much prehospital care, and did not receive much.

2. ANS—B *PEC—6*

Dr. J. Frank Pantridge, a cardiologist at the Royal Victoria Hospital in Belfast, Northern Ireland, introduced the concept of bringing advanced cardiac life support to the patient in the field. His paper titled: "A Mobile Intensive Care Unit" established the basis for future prehospital efforts.

3. ANS—B *PEC—6*

Dr. Eugene Nagel, of the University of Miami School of Medicine, trained a group of Miami Firefighters to be the first paramedics. He developed the first telemetry unit from an old milk crate and was the first to extend his medical license to paraprofessionals in the field. Since then, formal training programs have been organized nationwide. Today over 400 paramedic training programs exist in the United States.

4. ANS—A *PEC—6-9*

Ethics are the rules of conduct that govern members of a particular group or profession. Examples of ethical codes for EMS include the EMT Code of Ethics, and the EMT Oath. They are not laws, or morals, but rather guidelines for proper behavior expected from professionals.

5. ANS—D *PEC—9*

Professionalism describes the conduct or qualities that characterize a practitioner in a particular field or occupation. Professionals take pride in their work and earn the respect of their peers by the way they conduct daily business. They are the role models who set high standards for themselves and their colleagues. The professional paramedic promotes only excellent quality patient care.

6. ANS—C *PEC—10*

On-scene duties of the paramedic include size-up and assuring scene safety; needs determination; communication; patient assessment; assigning priorities of care; developing a treatment plan; leading the patient care team; initiating basic and advanced life support procedures; assessing the effects of treatment; establishing contact with the medical control physician; directing and coordinating patient transportation; and maintaining rapport with patients, support agencies, and hospital personnel. Maintaining current certification is an off-duty responsibility.

7. ANS—B *PEC—12*

Certification is the process by which an agency or association grants recognition to an individual who has met its qualifications. It is not a license to practice, but rather a statement that a person has fulfilled predetermined requirements. Each paramedic must maintain current certification by following the guidelines established by the certifying agency.

8. ANS—A   *PEC—13*

A license is permission to engage in a given occupation. A governmental agency grants licensure to individuals who have attained the degree of competency required to ensure the public's protection. A state grants a license to teachers, physicians, nurses, and barbers. Some states also license their paramedics.

9. ANS—C   *PEC—13*

Reciprocity is the process by which an agency grants automatic certification or licensure to an individual who has comparable credentials from another agency. Some states grant automatic paramedic certification to a person who holds a paramedic card from another state. Others grant certification to individuals who are nationally registered.

10. ANS—A   *PEC—13*

Belonging to a national EMS organization is an excellent way to communicate with members from other parts of the country. Some national organizations include the National Association for Search and Rescue (NASAR), the National Association of EMS Physicians (NAEMSP), and the National Association of EMT's (NAEMT).

11. ANS—D   *PEC—14*

The National Registry is an agency that prepares and administers standardized testing materials; assists in developing and evaluating training programs; establishes the qualifications for registration; and serves as a major tool for reciprocity by establishing the national minimum standard for competency.

12. ANS—B   *PEC—14*

Professional paramedics spend the vast majority of their time preparing for the next emergency call. Being a paramedic means accepting the responsibility of being the leader in the prehospital phase of emergency medical care. Leaders understand that the key to performance is preparation. The end of the training program marks only the beginning of the paramedic's education.

CHAPTER 2

Emergency Medical Services Systems

QUESTIONS

1. The type of EMS system in which various levels of responders are dispatched to calls depending on the severity of the situation is known as a
A. multi-level system
B. standard sytem
C. call screening system
D. tiered system

2. In 1966, the "White Paper"
A. deleted all federal funding for EMS
B. outlined deficiencies in emergency care
C. established the "15 components" of an EMS system
D. appropriated over $200 million dollars for EMS

3. Which of the following was **NOT** a necessary requirement to receive federal dollars from the EMS Systems Act of 1973?
A. Training
B. Mutual aid
C. Consumer participation
D. Medical direction

4. State EMS agencies are usually responsible for all of the following **EXCEPT**
A. contracting local medical directors
B. enacting EMS legislation

    C. licensing and certifying field personnel

    D. enforcing statewide EMS regulations

5. Who has the ultimate authority in all patient care-related issues in a local EMS system?

    A. State EMS Director

    B. System Medical Director

    C. Chief Paramedic on-duty

    D. Local EMS Coordinator

6. Which of the following is an example of direct medical control?

    A. Developing protocols and standing orders

    B. Consulting with the physician on radio during an emergency call

    C. Designing Continuing Quality Improvement activities

    D. Conducting chart reviews

7. Paramedic field interventions that are completed before contacting the medical control physician are known as

    A. indirect medical control orders

    B. the 4 "Ts"

    C. intervener physician protocols

    D. standing orders

8. Which of the following are important areas in which to educate the public?

    A. How to easily access the EMS system

    B. How to initiate basic life support procedures

    C. How to recognize a medical emergency

    D. All of the above

9. Which of the following is a component of a modern E-911 system?

    A. Instant call-back capabilities

    B. Automatic caller location

    C. Instant routing of the call

    D. All of the above

10. A system of emergency medical dispatching introduced by the Salt Lake City Fire Department that standardizes every aspect of dispatching emergency vehicles is known as

    A. priority dispatching

    B. pre-arrival dispatching

    C. triage dispatching

    D. call screening

11. System status management determines ambulance placement based on

    A. projected call volumes and locations

    B. signed contracts

    C. political sectors

    D. geographical boundaries

12. Which of the following is a nationally recognized level of EMT?

    A. EMT—Critical Care

    B. EMT—Ambulance

C. EMT—Intermediate

D. EMT—Cardiac Technician

13. Which governmental agency develops training curricula for all EMT training programs?

A. Department of Education

B. Department of Transportation

C. Department of Health and Human Services

D. Department of Public Safety

14. In 1983, the American College of Surgeons established guidelines for

A. ambulance specifications

B. response times for trauma

C. BLS equipment to be carried in ambulances

D. the use of the pneumatic antishock garment

15. The KKK standards deal with

A. ambulance safety and design

B. minimum standard medical protocols

C. training and education of field personnel

D. air evacuation of trauma victims

16. In 1970, the MAST program was established to

A. raise the blood pressure in shock victims

B. bring military air medical transport capabilities to civilian accident scenes

C. lower the evacuation times for wounded soldiers in Vietnam

D. to raise funds to establish regional EMS systems

17. Research in EMS is important in order to

A. justify future funding allocations

B. scientifically evaluate paramedical care

C. weigh the benefits versus the risks of certain prehospital treatments

D. all of the above

18. Hospital categorization is important because

A. not every patient can afford every hospital

B. receiving facilities have varying capabilities

C. not all patients can be transported to the appropriate facility

D. it is impossible to match patient needs with hospital resources

19. Quality assurance differs from quality improvement in that

A. quality assurance deals with patient perceptions of quality

B. quality improvement is an objective look at clinical care

C. quality assurance is often viewed as punitive and negative

D. quality improvement does not ellicit customer satisfaction information

20. The Public Utility Model and the Failsafe Franchise are examples of

A. CQI programs

B. KKK standards

C. system financing

D. dispatching protocols

ANSWERS **1. ANS—D** *PEC—19*

A "tiered" system is one in which basic life support first responders are dispatched unless advanced life support is needed. In that case, both are simultaneously dispatched to the emergency and the first responders initiate care until the higher level arrives.

2. ANS—B *PEC—20*

In 1966, the National Academy of Sciences—National Research Council published a paper titled: "Accidental Death and Disability, the Neglected Disease of Modern Society." The "White Paper," as it is better known, focused national attention on the problem of inadequate emergency medical care. It suggested guidelines for developing regional EMS systems, training prehospital care providers, and upgrading ambulances and their equipment. This landmark publication set off a series of federal and private funding initiatives.

3. ANS—D *PEC—21*

Of the 15 necessary components, the two that are missing are the most interesting. The authors of this legislation never foresaw the need to ensure medical direction and physician involvement in EMS system design. Neither did they see the need to ensure the financial stability of these programs in the event that the "soft" federal dollars became scarce. Both of these oversights led EMS in the wrong direction.

4. ANS—A *PEC—22*

State EMS agencies are typically responsible for: allocating funding to local systems; acting legislation concerning the prehospital practice of medicine; licensing and certifying field providers; enforcing all State EMS regulations; and appointing regional advisory councils. Hiring a local system medical director is the responsibility of the local EMS administrative agency.

5. ANS—B *PEC—22*

The local EMS system medical director is the ultimate authority in all patient care-related issues in the local EMS system. All prehospital patient care activities are extensions of this physician's license. Only a physician is licensed to practice medicine. This doctrine is known as "delegation of authority."

6. ANS—B *PEC—23*

Direct medical control exists when prehospital providers communicate directly with the physician at a medical control or Resource hospital. The physician's direction is usually based on established protocols from managing specific problems. This physician assumes responsibility and gives treatment orders for patients. Direct medical control physicians should be experienced in emergency medicine.

7. ANS—D *PEC—24*

Paramedic field interventions that are completed before contacting the medical control physician are known as standing orders. Standing orders are established by indirect medical control prior to the emergency call. These allow paramedics to perform certain procedures without a direct order from the base station physician.

8. ANS—D *PEC—25*

The public is an essential but often overlooked component of an EMS system.

An EMS system should have a plan for educating the public about recognizing an emergency situation, accessing the EMS system, and initiating basic life support procedures.

9. ANS—D   *PEC—25*

The basic emergency telephone number, 911, is a toll-free telephone service that enables the caller to dial three digits to reach a single public safety answering point. Enhanced 911 gives automatic location of the caller, instant routing of the call to the appropriate emergency service agency, and instant call back capabilities if the caller hangs up too soon.

10. ANS—A   *PEC—27*

A system of emergency medical dispatching introduced by the Salt Lake City Fire Department that standardizes every aspect of dispatching emergency vehicles is known as priority dispatching. In this system, medical dispatchers are trained to medically interrogate the distressed caller, prioritize symptoms, select the appropriate response, and give life-saving pre-arrival instructions. These protocols are designed and approved by the system medical director.

11. ANS—A   *PEC—26*

System status management is an emergency medical dispatching tool used to place ambulances and crews strategically around an EMS coverage area. The system status manager relies on projected call volumes and locations rather than geographical or political traditions. It is used to reduce response times.

12. ANS—C   *PEC—28*

The National Registry of EMTs recognizes and the Department of Transportation develops training curricula for three levels of field providers: EMT-Basic, EMT-Intermediate, and EMT-Paramedic. There exist, however, approximately 30 various levels of field provider nationwide.

13. ANS—B   *PEC—28*

Training curricula for EMT training programs are developed by the United States Department of Transportation. In 1966, Congress passed the National Highway Safety Act which forced the states to develop regional EMS systems or risk losing federal highway construction funds. The Department of Transportation was entrusted with developing the training curricula for these programs.

14. ANS—C   *PEC—29*

In 1983 the American College of Surgeons Committee on Trauma recommended a standard set of equipment to be carried by providers of basic life support services. In 1988, the American College of Emergency Physicians published a recommended list of advanced life support supplies and equipment to be carried on ALS units. Both sets of recommendations serve as excellent guidelines for any prehospital EMS system.

15. ANS—A   *PEC—29*

In 1974 responding to a request from the Department of Transportation, the General Services Administration developed the KKK standards, which established federal specifications for ambulances. The original guidelines and the subsequent revisions were aimed at improving ambulance design and safety features.

16. ANS—B *PEC—31*

In 1970, the Military Assistance to Safety and Traffic (MAST) program was established. This demonstration project set up 35 programs nationwide to test the feasibility of using military helicopters and paramedical personnel in civilian medical emergencies.

17. ANS—D *PEC—34*

In order to provide a scientific basis for prehospital EMS, a formal ongoing research program is an essential component of the system. Research is necessary to justify future funding allocations, to scientifically evaluate paramedical care, and to weigh the benefits versus the risks of certain prehospital treatments.

18. ANS—B *PEC—34*

Since all hospitals are not all equal in emergency and support service capabilities hospital categorization is an important component of an EMS system. It identifies the readiness and capability of a hospital and its staff to receive and effectively treat emergency patients. Categorization originated from the realization that patients have varying degrees of illness and injury and that receiving facilities have varying capabilities to provide initial or definitive care.

19. ANS—C *PEC—32*

Quality assurance programs are primarily designed to maintain continuous monitoring and measurement of the quality of clinical care delivered. They emphasize evaluation of response times, adherence to protocols, patient survival, and other indicators. They are often viewed as punitive and negative.

20. ANS—C *PEC—36*

The public utility model and the fail safe franchise are examples of system financing. In these systems municipalities establish the design and standards for the contract bid and periodically, usually every three or four years, hold wholesale competition for the market.

CHAPTER 3

Medical Legal Considerations in Emergency Care

QUESTIONS

1. Homocide and rape are examples of wrongs against society and would be tried in
   A. criminal court
   B. tort court
   C. civil court
   D. none of the above

2. Which of the following would be an example of a tort case?
   A. Divorce
   B. Suicide
   C. Contract dispute
   D. Malpractice

3. Paramedics could find themselves involved in which types of legal cases?
   A. Tort cases
   B. Civil cases
   C. Criminal cases
   D. All of the above

4. A "Medical Practice Act"
   A. defines the scope of practice for allied health care professionals
   B. is a national standard for allied health care professionals

     C. outlines ethical behavior guidelines for medical paraprofessionals
     D. is unecessary in states that license their paramedics

5. The doctrine of "delegation of authority" states that
     A. paramedics may practice independently
     B. paramedics may only practice under the license of a physician
     C. paramedics cannot be found criminally liable for practicing without a license
     D. paramedics do not require a "Medical Practice Act"

6. Laws that protect health care workers from liability in the event they stop and render roadside care are known as
     A. Good Samaritan Laws
     B. *Res ipsa loquitor* laws
     C. Delegation of Authority laws
     D. Negligence laws

7. If a question arises concerning the validity of "Do Not Resuscitate" orders or "Living Wills," the paramedic should
     A. contact medical control
     B. ignore all such orders and run the code
     C. accept and honor all such orders
     D. run a "slow code" in these cases

8. Negligence is defined as
     A. lawsuits involving no physical harm
     B. deviating from the standard of care
     C. failing to prove proximate cause
     D. all of the above

9. Which of the following is **NOT** a necessary component of a successful negligence suit?
     A. Duty to act
     B. Breach of duty
     C. Proximate cause
     D. Unlawful consent

10. In *res ipsa loquitor*, the burden of proof rests with the
     A. plaintiff
     B. defendant
     C. medical advisory council
     D. district attorney

11. Informed consent means
     A. the adult patient is mentally competent
     B. the patient understands the treatment and the risks
     C. the patient agrees to the treatment
     D. all of the above

12. Which of the following would **NOT** fall under the concept of implied consent?
     A. An unconscious diabetic in insulin shock
     B. A 5-year-old in anaphylactic shock with no parent present

    C. A mentally retarded person with bilateral fractured femurs

    D. A diabetic who awakens following 50% Dextrose therapy and refuses transport

13. Failure to formally transfer the patient to medical staff in the emergency department could place the paramedic in danger of being sued for

    A. false imprisonment

    B. unlawful consent

    C. abandonment

    D. patient endangerment

14. Threatening to defibrillate a patient if he does not quiet down could place a paramedic in danger of being sued for

    A. assault

    B. battery

    C. libel

    D. slander

15. Starting an IV on a competent patient who absolutely refuses one could place the paramedic in danger of being sued for

    A. assault

    B. battery

    C. libel

    D. slander

16. Transporting a patient to the hospital against his will could place the paramedic in danger of being sued for

    A. false imprisonment

    B. kidnapping

    C. unlawful consent

    D. assault and battery

17. Stating on the air that "We've got Frank Ashby again, and he's drunk and obnoxious as usual" could place the paramedic in danger of being sued for

    A. assault

    B. battery

    C. libel

    D. slander

18. Writing on the run sheet that a certain patient "probably has AIDS from deviant homosexual activity" could place the paramedic in danger of being sued for

    A. assault

    B. definition of character

    C. libel

    D. slander

19. Which of the following statements is true concerning prehospital documentation?

    A. If you don't write it down, you did not do it

    B. A well documented run sheet can be your best defense in court

    C. Intentional alterations of the run sheet are considered admissions of guilt

    D. All of the above

20. A paramedic's best defense against potential legal liability is

    A. purchasing medical malpractice insurance

    B. documenting as little as possible on the run sheet

    C. relying on Good Samaritan immunity

    D. practicing excellent quality prehospital care

ANSWERS

1. ANS—A *PEC—41*

Criminal law deals with crimes against society and their punishments. Criminal litigations are legal actions taken by the state against the offending individual. Homocide and rape are examples of criminal wrongs. To convict requires proof beyond a reasonable doubt.

2. ANS—D *PEC—41*

Tort law, a branch of civil law, deals with civil wrongs committed by one individual against another. A medical malpractice suit is an example of tort against a paramedic. Unlike a criminal case, only a preponderance of evidence (50% +1) is needed to win the case.

3. ANS—D *PEC—41*

Paramedics may become involved in any aspect of the legal system. They may be called as witnesses in a criminal offense, asked to testify in a civil matter, or named in malpractice litigation.

4. ANS—A *PEC—41*

A "Medical Practice Act" is specific state legislation that defines the scope and role of the paramedic and other allied health care professionals. It establishes the requirements for those who will be allowed to practice and identifies certification and licensing procedures. Medical Practice acts differ from state to state.

5. ANS—B *PEC—41*

Paramedics are not licensed to practice independently. They may only function under the supervision of a licensed physician through delegation of authority. This supervision may be direct (in person, on radio) or indirect (protocols, standing orders). Failure to adhere to this requirement could make the paramedic criminally liable for practicing medicine without a license. In some states, this constititues a felony, punishable by fines or imprisonment.

6. ANS—A *PEC—41*

Laws which protect off-duty health care workers from liability in the event they stop and render roadside care are known as Good Samaritan Laws. A person is immune from liability for assisting at the scene of a medical emergency if he or she acts in good faith, is not grossly negligent, and does not accept payment for services. Unfortunately, gross negligence is a subjective term and the plaintiff's attorney will portray the paramedic as such. A jury of non-medical civilians will listen to testimony and decide the outcome. In many cases, the Good Samaritan defense has not held up in court.

7. ANS—A *PEC—42*

When questions concerning the validity of "Do Not Resuscitate" orders or "Living Wills" arise in the field, paramedics should contact medical control. Paramedics don't have the legal authority and are not in the position to evaluate the validity of such documents.

8. ANS—B *PEC—44*

Negligence is defined as deviating from accepted standards of care. In medicine, negligence is synonymous with malpractice. Paramedics can be negligent by not performing to the standard of care (failing to immobilize the c-spine); by performing beyond their training and certification (any skill not approved by the local medical director); or by substandard performance (unrecognized esophageal intubation of a breathing patient).

9. ANS—D *PEC—44*

To win a negligence case the plaintiff's attorney must prove that a paramedic's breach of duty caused harm to the patient. Once again, in a tort case, only a preponderance of evidence is needed to win.

10. ANS—B *PEC—44*

When the doctrine of *res ipsa loquitor* is invoked, the burden of proof shifts from the plantiff to the defendant. *Res ipsa loquitor* is latin for "things speaks for itself" and states that the damages could not have occurred in the absence of the paramedic's negligence. For example, only the paramedic could have placed the endotracheal tube into the esophagus.

11. ANS—D *PEC—45*

Informed consent must be obtained from every conscious, mentally competent adult person before treatment can be started. Informed consent means that the adult patient is mentally competent, understands the treatment and the risks, and agrees to be treated.

12. ANS—D *PEC—45*

Unconscious patients cannot express consent. When treating the unconscious patient the treatment is considered to be implied. With implied consent it is assumed that the patient would want life-saving treatment if he or she were able to provide expressed consent.

13. ANS—C *PEC—46*

Abandonment is the termination of the paramedic-patient relationship without assuring a mechanism for the continuation of the care. Paramedics should not initiate care and then arbitrarily discontinue it. Physically leaving a patient unattended on an emergency department stretcher may be grounds for abandonment if the patient's condition deteriorates.

14. ANS—A *PEC—46*

Assault is defined as unlawfully placing a person in apprehension of immediate bodily harm without his or her consent. Threatening to defibrillate a patient if he does not quiet down could place a paramedic in danger of being sued for assault. Assault can be either a criminal or a civil offense.

15. ANS—B *PEC—46*

Battery is the unlawful touching of another individual without his or her consent. Starting an IV on a competent patient who absolutely refuses one could place the paramedic in danger of being sued for battery. Battery could also be a criminal or a civil offense.

16. ANS—A   *PEC—46*

Everyone has the right to be left alone. False imprisonment is defined as unlawful and unjustifiable detention. Transporting a patient to the hospital against his will could constitute false imprisonment. In these cases, paramedics should ensure that the transportation is medically justified.

17. ANS—D   *PEC—47*

Slander is the act of injuring a person's character, name, or reputation by false or malicious spoken words. Information transmitted over the radio should be limited to essential matters of patient care. The medical report should never contain the patient's name or the paramedic's subjective opinions.

18. ANS—C   *PEC—47*

Libel is the act of injuring a person's character, name, or reputation by false or malicious writings. Alligations of libel can be avoided by respecting the patient's confidentiality. The medical record should be accurate and confidential, slang and labels should be avoided. Never write anything on the run report that could be construed as libel.

19. ANS—D   *PEC—48*

A complete well written run report is a paramedic's best protection in a malpractice proceeding. To the court, observations and treatments not documented on the run report were not performed. The medical records should never be altered, as it amounts to an admission of guilt by the paramedic.

20. ANS—D   *PEC—48*

A paramedic's best defense against potential legal liability is practicing the highest quality of patient care, which includes good documentation.

CHAPTER 4

EMS Communications

QUESTIONS

1. The principle transmitter and receiver of a communications system is known as the
A. mobile radio
B. base station
C. satellite
D. repeater

2. Which of the following will **NOT** impede the range of radio transmissions?
A. Flatlands
B. Mountains
C. High buildings
D. Dense foliage

3. A device that receives a transmission from a low-power source on one frequency and retransmits it at a higher power on another frequency is a/an
A. mobile transmitter
B. repeater
C. encoder
D. decoder

4. The process by which low power transmissions are selected by the

receiver that picks up the strongest signal and boosts the signal to the base station is known as
A. decoding
B. boosting
C. encoding
D. voting

5. A device that transmits specific tones to activate certain radios is called a/an
A. encoder
B. voter
C. repeater
D. decoder

6. A radio pager is an example of a/an
A. encoder
B. decoder
C. repeater
D. voter

7. Which of the following is an advantage of using cellular communications?
A. 12 lead ECGs can be transmitted
B. FAX and computer messages can be transmitted
C. Dedicated paramedic lines can be established
D. All of the above

8. A group of radio frequencies close together is called a
A. band
B. spectrum
C. multiplex
D. UHF configuration

9. Which of the following is not an EMS frequency range?
A. VHF-Lo
B. VHF-High
C. UHF
D. AM

10. Which of the following radio frequency ranges offers the clearest communications with the least interference?
A. 30–50 MHz
B. 150–170 MHz
C. 450–470 MHz
D. 800+ MHz

11. Trunking is a communications term that describes
A. computerized frequency allocation
B. hard-wiring for ambulance radios
C. base station radio procedues
D. multiple antennae installation

12. Which of the "med channels" are designated for paramedic to physician communications?

    A. 1–8

    B. 9–10

    C. All 10

    D. 1–2

13. Transmitting the patient's ECG over the air is a process known as

    A. demodulation

    B. voting

    C. biotelemetry

    D. trunking

14. A modulator

    A. converts radio tones into ECG voltage changes

    B. converts ECG voltage changes into radio tones

    C. is found in the hospital base station

    D. displays its signal on an oscilloscope

15. Which of the following can cause ECG interference?

    A. Loose electrodes

    B. Muscle tremors

    C. 60 Hz

    D. All of the above

16. In which type of communications system does transmission and reception occur on the same frequency?

    A. Simplex

    B. Duplex

    C. Multiplex

    D. Biotelemetry

17. In which type of communications system can transmission and reception occur simultaneously?

    A. Simplex

    B. Duplex

    C. Multiplex

    D. Biotelemetry

18. In which type of communications system can biotelemetry information be transmitted during conversation on the same frequency?

    A. Simplex

    B. Duplex

    C. Multiplex

    D. Biotelemetry

19. Which of the following is true concerning radio equipment maintenance?

    A. Regular maintenance can improve the radio's life expectancy

    B. Cleaning solvents can be used on the outer case safely

    C. Any paramedic can perform simple repairs on the radio

    D. Simply dropping a radio rarely causes damage

20. The governmental agency that regulates all radio communications is the

    A. Department of Transportation

    B. Department of Communications

C. Federal Communications Commission
D. National Association of Broadcasting

ANSWERS

1. ANS—B   *PEC—54*

The principle transmitter and receiver of a communications system is known as the base station. It is usually the most powerful radio in the system with output typically 45-275 watts. Some base stations are multiple channel systems, but most can only communicate on one channel at a time.

2. ANS—A   *PEC—55*

Transmissions over flatland or water will not impede the range. Transmissions over mountains, through dense foilage, or in urban areas of large buildings will decrease the range.

3. ANS—B   *PEC—55*

A repeater is a device that receives a transmission from a low power portable or a mobile radio on one frequency and re-transmits it at a higher power on another frequency. Repeaters are important in large geographical areas because portable and mobile radios may not have enough range to communicate with each other, with medical control, or with the dispatcher.

4. ANS—D   *PEC—55*

Many large EMS systems have more than one repeater. Often, when a mobile unit transmits, more than one repeater will pick up the transmission. A system designed so that the repeater receiving the strongest signal will transmit the message is known as voting.

5. ANS—A   *PEC—56*

A device for generating unique codes or tones that are recognized by another radio's decoder is called an encoder. An encoder is similar to a telephone keypad. When activated by pressing the buttons, it sends specific tones over the air.

6. ANS—B   *PEC—56*

A device that receives and recognizes unique codes or tones sent over the air is called a decoder. Only the sequence of tones specific for that decoder will activate it. Most radio pagers work on this principle.

7. ANS—D   *PEC—57*

Many EMS systems are using cellular communications. Advantages include: the ability to transmit 12 lead EKGs, fax, and computer messages, and the ability to establish dedicated paramedic lines into the base station hospital.

8. ANS—A   *PEC—58*

A group of radio frequencies close together on the electromagnetic spectrum is called a band. Some examples of radio bands are AM, FM, citizen band, short wave, UHF, and VHF.

9. ANS—D   *PEC—58*

The FCC has designated certain bands for use in EMS. They include VHF low, 30-50 MHz; VHF high, 150-170 MHz; UHF 450-470 MHz, and a new band in the 800 MHz range.

10. ANS—D   *PEC—58*

As a rule, the lower the band the farther the range, but the more interference. The clearest communications in EMS can be utilized in the 800 megahertz range UHF. UHF transmissions have less range than VHF, but they are less susceptable to interference.

11. ANS—A   *PEC—58*

In a trunked system, all frequencies are pooled together. A computer routs a radio transmission to the first available frequency. All subsequent transmissions are routed in the same manner. This eliminates the need to search for unused frequencies.

12. ANS—A   *PEC—59*

The FCC has designated EMS channels for use nationwide on the UHF band. Channels 1-8 are designated for paramedic to physician communications. Channels 9-10 are for dispatching purposes.

13. ANS—C   *PEC—59*

The process of transmitting physiological data such as an ECG over distance, usually by radio, is known as biotelemetry. An example of this is the paramedic transmitting the ECG over the air to the base station physician in the hospital.

14. ANS—B   *PEC—59*

A device that tranforms electrical energy into sound waves is known as a modulator. The patient's biotelemetry radio is an example of a modulator. It transforms the patient's ECG voltage changes into radio tones, which are then transmitted to the hospital.

Figure 4-1

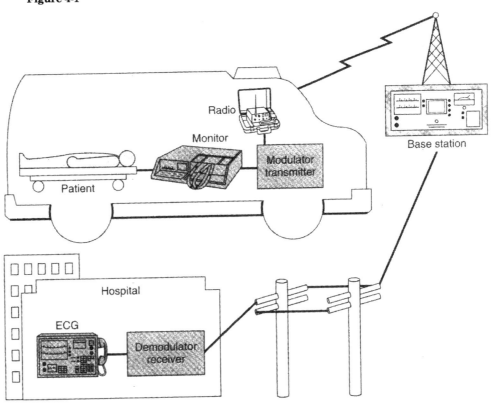

Source: PEC, Figure 4–12.

15. ANS—D   *PEC—60*

Biotelemetry communications are subject to interference by such things as muscle tremors, loose electrodes, 60 hertz interference, fluctuations in transmitter power, and by the transmission of voice communications while telemetry is in progress.

16. ANS—A   *PEC—60*

In a simplex system, transmission and reception cannot occur at the same time because they both occur on the same frequency. A person must transmit a message, release the button, and wait for a response.

Figure 4-2

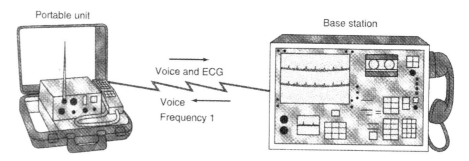

Source: PEC, Figure 4–13.

17. ANS—B   *PEC—60*

In duplex systems, two frequencies are used much like telephone communications. This means that transmission and reception can occur at the same time.

Figure 4-3

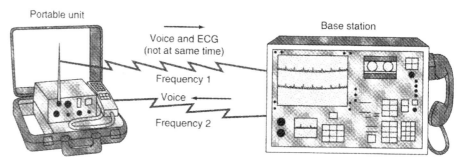

Source: PEC, Figure 4–14.

18. ANS—C *PEC—61*

In multiplex systems, radio transmission and other data such as EKG can be transmitted simultaneously by the use of multiple frequencies.

Figure 4-4

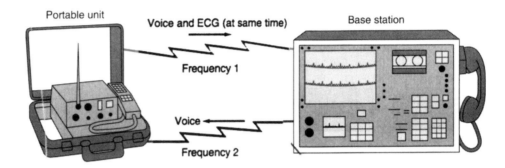

Source: PEC, Figure 4–15.

19. ANS—A *PEC—61*

Radio equipment is expensive and fragile. A regular schedule of maintenance and cleaning will improve its appearance and life expectancy. Careful handling can increase its longevity and improve its performance.

20. ANS—C *PEC—61*

The Federal Communications Commission is the governmental agency responsible for assigning frequencies, regulating all radios, and controlling all radio communications in the United States.

CHAPTER 5

Rescue Operations

SCENARIO You are called to the scene of a partial building collapse caused by a minor earthquake where one victim is trapped under some debris. Reports from the scene verify the need for a heavy search and rescue operation. You are the paramedic in charge of patient care. Upon arrival at the scene, you meet the Fire Department Rescue Officer and begin discussing the operation. Part of the building has indeed collapsed and the uncollapsed portions appear to be unstable.

1. The highest priority in any rescue situation is
   A. patient care
   B. rescuer safety
   C. time management
   D. extrication

2. The decision whether to attempt or not to attempt a dangerous rescue should be made by the
   A. rescue captain
   B. fire chief
   C. safety officer
   D. paramedic in charge

3. Which of the following is included in the screening criteria for rescue personnel?
  A. Psychological testing
  B. Physical capabilities
  C. Phobia testing
  D. All of the above

4. The paramedic's responsibilities in a rescue operation include
  A. assessing the patient as soon as possible
  B. maintaining patient care throughout disentanglement
  C. accompanying the patient during removal and transport
  D. all of the above

5. Which of the following foods are recommended for extended rescue operations?
  A. Complex carbohydrates and water
  B. Cookies and milk
  C. Coffee and doughnuts
  D. Soda and pretzels

6. Which of the following is included in the rescue assessment?
  A. Nature of the situation
  B. Number of victims
  C. Scene hazards
  D. All of the above

7. Which of the following may be helpful during this rescue operation?
  A. Search dogs
  B. Electronic detection devices
  C. Experienced search managers
  D. All of the above

8. Which of the following typically results in a poorly executed rescue operation?
  A. Undertrained personnel
  B. Poorly equipped personnel
  C. Not knowing what team members are doing
  D. All of the above

9. Guidelines for managing patients with prolonged exposure are published by the
  A. Wilderness Medical Society
  B. Wilderness EMT course
  C. National Association for Search and Rescue
  D. all of the above

10. Which of the following would be helpful in providing psychological support for this victim?
  A. Avoid using his name
  B. Do not introduce yourself
  C. Explain all delays in the rescue operation
  D. Never describe the technical aspects of the operation

ANSWERS

1. ANS—B
PEC—70

Your own personal safety is your first and major concern in any rescue situation.

2. ANS—C
PEC—73

The safety officer is the person with the knowledge and authority to intervene in an unsafe rescue situation. This person should make all go / no-go decisions for every rescue operation.

3. ANS—D
PEC—73

Search and rescue teams often use personnel screening to determine who may participate in a rescue process. Programs are available that identify physical capabilities of crew members. In addition, psychological testing and phobia screening may even be desirable.

4. ANS—D
PEC—78

In a rescue situation the paramedic has three major responsibilities: initiating patient assessment and care as soon as possible; maintaining patient care procedures throughout disentanglement; and accompanying the patient during removal and transport.

5. ANS—A
PEC—74

Predetermined policies regarding food and hydration are an important part of the rescue preplan. To maintain maximum personnel performance rescuers should eat frequently but in small amounts. The diet should be high in complex carbohydrates, low in sugars and fats. Fluid replacement should consist of plain water or relatively dilute electrolyte solutions.

6. ANS—D
PEC—75

The rescue assessment begins with the dispatchers call and your subsequent arrival at the scene. It is necessary to evaluate the nature of the situation, any on-scene hazards, specific patient location, and the number of victims involved.

7. ANS—D
PEC—76

On rare occasions you will come across rescue situations like this that hide patients. If possible, ask your dispatcher to send an on-scene specialist to meet the crew. Search dogs, electronic detection devices, or experienced search managers may also be required.

8. ANS—D
PEC—77

Poorly executed rescue operations are usually caused by undertrained and poorly equipped personnel. Also team members frequently do not know what other team members are doing.

9. ANS—D
PEC—79

Position papers of the Wilderness Medical Society or the Wilderness EMT Course, sponsored by the National Association for Search and Rescue, can serve as guidelines for protocols that anticipate prolonged patient care situations.

10. ANS—C
PEC—80

In order to provide more indepth psychological support for rescue patients in a prolonged extrication operation you should do the following:

- Learn and use the patient's name.

- Be sure the patient knows your name and that you will not abandon him or her.

- Be sure that other team members know and use the patient's correct name.

- Avoid negative comments regarding the operation or the patient's condition within ear shot of the patient.

- Explain all delays to the patient and reassure him or her if problems arise.

- Ask special rescue teams to explain technical aspects of the operation that could directly impact the patient's condition. Translate these operations into clear, simple terms for the patient.

CHAPTER 6

Major Incident Response

QUESTIONS

SCENARIO You are dispatched to a possible multiple patient incident involving a derailed train. Initial reports indicate two derailed passenger cars with approximately 30–50 victims still inside. Fire department rescue crews are busy with search operations and extrication procedures. As you approach the scene, you are designated officer of the medical sector. You are responsible for all medical aspects of this incident.

1. The level of intensity of this incident indicates a
   A. Level I response
   B. Level II response
   C. Level III response
   D. Level IV response

2. Advantages of using the Incident Command System include
   A. providing an organizational plan
   B. identifying lines of authority
   C. providing a means for processing information
   D. all of the above

3. Incident command should be established
   A. when top ranking officers arrive
   B. when the fire department arrives

C. when law enforcement arrives

D. when the first unit arrives

4. An orderly transfer of command process includes

    A. face-to-face communication

    B. a radio announcement

    C. a formal briefing

    D. all of the above

5. In order to avoid congestion at the scene it is useful to

    A. stage vehicles at a central location until needed at the scene

    B. only request the number of vehicles you absolutely need

    C. limit responding units to a minimum

    D. have responding units park away from the scene and send only personnel in

6. The sector normally assigned to work in the hazard zone is

    A. triage

    B. treatment

    C. extrication

    D. supply

7. Locating and removing victims from the hazard zone is the responsibility of the

    A. extrication sector

    B. treatment sector

    C. triage sector

    D. transportation sector

8. Providing a safe area to collect patients once removed from the hazard zone is the responsibility of the

    A. extrication sector

    B. treatment sector

    C. triage sector

    D. staging sector

9. Establishing an ambulance loading zone is the responsibility of the

    A. staging sector

    B. treatment sector

    C. triage sector

    D. transportation sector

10. Collecting resources at a central site to avoid scene congestion is the responsibility of the

    A. supply sector

    B. treatment sector

    C. staging sector

    D. transportation sector

11. Coordinating supplies to be used in the treatment area is the responsibility of the

    A. extrication sector

    B. treatment sector

    C. triage sector

    D. supply sector

12. As you encounter walking wounded you should
    A. move them to the treatment area
    B. ignore them
    C. move them to an area other than the treatment area
    D. transport them immediately

Indicate whether you would categorize the following patients as Immediate or Delayed:

13. 56-year-old male bleeding from a scalp laceration, respiratory rate of 26, radial pulse, acts confused and disoriented.

14. 23-year-old female with abdominal pain, respirations 20, radial pulse, alert and oriented.

15. 25-year-old male with abdominal pain and guarding, respiratory rate 28, no radial pulse, disoriented.

16. 35-year-old with unstable flail chest, respirations 36, radial pulse, alert.

17. 78-year-old with fractured humerus, respirations 20, radial pulse, alert.

18. Within sectors what type of communication is recommended?
    A. Portable radios
    B. Mobile radios
    C. Face-to-face
    D. None of the above

19. In this communications system who is allowed to talk with the incident commander?
    A. Anyone who needs to
    B. People at the command post only
    C. Sector officers
    D. All arriving units

20. Which of the following items are beneficial at a major incident?
    A. Sector vests
    B. Pencils
    C. Worksheets
    D. All of the above

ANSWERS   **1. ANS—B**   *PEC—88*

The EMS response to a multiple casualty incident can be divided into three categories based upon the resources required at the scene. This particular incident requires a Level II response in that it will overwhelm the a local EMS system and rescue personnel. A Level II incident typically involves a large number of patients and may involve more than one incident site. Often it may include overlapping jurisdictional boundaries requiring inter-agency coordination. A Level II response usually necessitates mutual aid from several outside agencies.

2. ANS—D   *PEC—90*

The benefits of using an incident command system include:

- Providing an organizational plan that is designed to manage incident needs effectively
- Providing a blueprint for organizing, controlling, and coordinating the substantial resources that are likely to respond to a major incident
- Providing an organizational framework in which similar functions are grouped
- Identifying and defining responsibilities and lines of authority
- Providing an orderly means to communicate and process information for decision making
- Providing a common terminology
- Identifying a transfer of command process
- Offering performance evaluation criteria

3. ANS—D   *PEC—90*

The basic principle of the incident command system is that overall incident command responsibilities be fixed on one person. This system further requires that a strong, direct, and visible command mode be established as early as possible during the operation, preferably by the first arriving unit.

4. ANS—D   *PEC—94*

An orderly transfer of command process includes face-to-face communication with a formal briefing and/or a radio announcement.

5. ANS—A   *PEC—91*

Staging describes the collecting of vehicles at a central location for distribution as needed at a major incident scene. It is used to avoid scene congestion.

6. ANS—C   *PEC—95*

The first sector usually established by the incident commander is the extrication sector. The extrication sector operates within the hazard zone.

7. ANS—A   *PEC—95*

Locating and removing victims from the hazard zone is a responsibility of the extrication sector.

Extrication Officer Responsibilities

1. Determine whether triage and primary treatment are to be conducted on site or at the treatment sector.
2. Determine resources needed to extricate trapped patients, and deliver them to the treatment sector.
3. Provide for site safety (very important!).
4. Determine resources needed for triage and primary treatment of patients.
5. Communicate resource requirements to command.
6. Allocate assigned resources.
7. Assign, direct, and supervise personnel and resources.
8. Collect, assemble, and assess patients with obvious minor injuries, and isolate them from the treatment and extrication sector operations.
9. Provide frequent progress reports to command.

> **10.** Report to command when all patients have been extricated and delivered to the treatment sector.
> **11.** Coordinate with other sectors as required.

8. ANS—B

PEC—97

Providing a safe area to collect patients once removed from the hazard zone is the responsibility of the treatment sector.

Treatment Officer Responsibilities

1. Locate a suitable treatment sector area, and report that location to the extrication sector manager and command.
2. Evaluate resources required for patient treatment, and report those needs to command.
3. Provide suitable "immediate" and "delayed" treatment areas.
4. Allocate resources.
5. Assign, direct, supervise, and coordinate personnel within the sector.
6. Report progress to command.
7. Coordinate with other sectors.

9. ANS—D

PEC—99

Establishing an ambulance loading zone is the responsibility of the transportation sector.

Transportation Officer Responsibilities

1. Establish ambulance staging (if command has not done so) and patient loading areas.
2. Establish and operate a helicopter landing site.
3. Work with the communication center and hospitals to obtain medical facility status and treatment capabilities.
4. Coordinate patient allocation and transportation with the treatment sector, the communication center, and hospitals.
5. Report resource requirements to command.
6. Supervise assigned personnel.
7. Coordinate with other sectors.
8. Report when the last patient has been transported.

10. ANS—C

PEC—101

Collecting resources at a central site to avoid scene congestion is the responsibility of the staging sector.

Staging Sector Officer Responsibilities

1. Coordinate with the police department to block streets, intersections, and other access routes required for staging operations.
2. Ensure that all apparatus and vehicles are parked in an appropriate and orderly manner within staging, so that they may be easily moved to the incident site.

3. Maintain a log of units available in the staging area, as well as an inventory of all specialized equipment and medical supplies that might be required at the scene.
4. Confer with command about essential resources in the staging area, and coordinate requests for these resources with the communications center.
5. Assume a position that is visible and accessible to incoming and staged units. This can best be accomplished by one unit leaving its emergency lights on, while all others turn their lights off upon entering the staging area. The staging officer will be located at the vehicle with its lights on. He or she should wear a sector vest.
6. Announce the location of staging to command and the communications center, so that all responding units will report to the proper staging location.

11. ANS—D   *PEC—101*

Coordinating supplies to be used in the treatment area is the responsibility of the supply sector.

Supply Sector Officer Responsibilities

1. Establish a suitable location for support sector operations, normally near the treatment sector.
2. Determine the medical supply and equipment needs of other sectors.
3. With the transportation sector, coordinate procurement of medical supplies from hospitals.
4. Coordinate the procurement of additional supplies that are not available from hospitals.
5. Report additional resource requirements to command.
6. Allocate supplies and equipment as needed.
7. Report progress to command.
8. Coordinate activities with other sectors.

12. ANS—C   *PEC—103*

The first on-scene rescuers clear the site of any walking wounded by verbally telling them to walk to a designated location. This location should be different from the treatment area and staffed with personnel to process them appropriately.

13. This patient's confusion and decreased mental status makes him Immediate.

14. This patient has no major respiratory, circulatory or neurological deficits and is Delayed.

15. This patient's absence of radial pulse and decreased mental status makes him Immediate.

16. This patient's respiratory rate of 36 makes her Immediate.

17. This patient has no major respiratory, circulatory, or neurological deficits and is Delayed.

18. ANS—C *PEC—104*

All personnel assigned to each sector work for and communicate only with their sector officer. In the vast majority of cases, because the sector officer is in the work area, this communication should be face-to-face.

19. ANS—C *PEC—104*

Under normal circumstances, only the sector officer should communicate with the incident commander.

20. ANS—D *PEC—106*

Sector vests are excellent tools in a rescue operation. These brightly colored garments identify sector officers in a crowd of rescuers. The need for documentation and patient tracking is obvious in a multi-casualty situation. You can develop pads or worksheets that organize important information and provide reminders of what needs to be done.

CHAPTER 7

Stress Management in Emergency Services

QUESTIONS

1. Which of the following statements is true regarding stress?
   A. It is a state of physical arousal
   B. It is a state of psychological arousal
   C. It exists to some degree in everyone
   D. All of the above

2. Any agent or situation that causes stress is called a/an
   A. antagonist
   B. stressor
   C. alarmist
   D. none of the above

3. Which of the following is **NOT** part of the body's response to stress?
   A. Release of epinephrine and norepinephrine
   B. The pulse rate and blood pressure decrease
   C. The pupils dilate
   D. Blood glucose levels increase

4. Which of the following best describes the alarm stage?
   A. It occurs at the first exposure to the stressor.
   B. It results in a sympathetic nervous system activation.
   C. If resistance is low, the response can be overwhelming.
   D. All of the above.

5. Which of the following best describes the resistance stage?
   A. The victim is beginning to cope.
   B. Vital signs return to normal.
   C. Resistance to stressor becomes stronger.
   D. All of the above

6. Which of the following best describes the exhaustion stage?
   A. The victim no longer can adapt to stressor.
   B. Alarm stage signs reappear.
   C. Alarm stage signs are more difficult to reverse.
   D. All of the above.

7. Which of the following statements is true regarding an acute stress reaction?
   A. It may occur during or immediately following a stressful incident.
   B. It may require immediate medical intervention
   C. It may require further psychological counselling
   D. All of the above

8. Which of the following statements is true regarding post-traumatic stress disorder?
   A. The symptoms may be physical, emotional, or behavioral.
   B. The symptoms may appear months or years following the incident.
   C. It may have a major negative influence on the rescuer's life.
   D. All of the above.

9. Which of the following statements best describes the term "burnout".
   A. Burnout is unavoidable in EMS.
   B. Burnout can be prevented.
   C. Burnout does not affect other aspects of the paramedic's life.
   D. Patient care rarely suffers as a result of paramedic burnout

10. Which of the following best describes anxiety?
   A. It is an emotional state
   B. It is caused by stress
   C. It results in an increase in sympathetic tone
   D. All of the above

11. Which of the following statements is true regarding stress?
   A. A certain amount of stress produces top performance
   B. Stress can help us cope with unusual stressors
   C. The body has the ability to adapt to stress
   D. All of the above

12. Which of the following is NOT a sign or symptom of stress?
   A. Heart palpitations
   B. GI distress
   C. Increased salivation
   D. Chest pain

13. Which of the following is NOT a physiological effect of stress?
   A. Deceased blood pressure
   B. Decreased circulation to the skin

C. Inceased blood glucose levels
D. Pupil dilation

14. Which of the following is a way to manage stress?
A. Solicit support from co-workers
B. Get adequate rest and sleep
C. Get involved in things outside of EMS
D. All of the above

15. Which of the following is **not** a definition of a Critical Incident Stress Debriefing?
A. It allows emergency personnel to discuss their feelings
B. It reduces the impact of a critical event
C. It accelerates the normal recovery of rescuers
D. It provides psychotherapy and psychological treatment

16. During the acceptance stage, the dying patient
A. is often devoid of feelings
B. is preparing to face death
C. is without fear and despair
D. all of the above

17. When informing someone of the death of a loved one, you should use the word
A. expired
B. passed away
C. dead
D. none of the above

18. During the anger stage
A. allow the patient and family to vent their feelings
B. understand their anger may be directed at you
C. don't take their remarks personally
D. all of the above

19. The dying patient who worries about who will make the funeral arrangements is an example of
A. reactive depression
B. preparatory depression
C. bargaining
D. none of the above

20. Which of the following best describes stress and paramedic life?
A. Stress is part of the EMS world
B. Paramedics must learn to deal with stress effectively
C. Too much stress can be physically and psychologically damaging
D. All of the above

ANSWERS **1. ANS—D** *PEC—112*

Stress is defined as a state of physical or psychological arousal that exists to some degree in everyone.

2. ANS—B *PEC—112*

Any agent or situation that causes stress is a stressor.

3. ANS—B *PEC—113*

As the body responds to stress, the endocrine system releases epinephrine and norepinephrine. These hormones cause increases in pulse and blood pressure (to deliver more oxygenated blood to vital organs), dilated pupils (to improve vision), excessive perspiration (to decrease body temperature), increased muscle tension (to anticipate increased muscle use), and increased blood glucose levels (to supply fuel to vital tissues).

4. ANS—D *PEC—113*

An alarm stage reaction occurs at the first exposure to the stressor. The signs include the normal responses of the sympathetic nervous stimulation (see answer 3). If the victim's resistance is lowered, the stress response may be overwhelming.

5. ANS—D *PEC—113*

The resistance stage begins as the victim adapts to the stressor. It is brought upon by the use of various coping mechanisms. Vital signs return to normal. As adaptation develops, resistance to the particular stressor increases.

6. ANS—D *PEC—113*

Prolonged exposure to the same stressors may lead to exhaustion of the victim's adaptation capabilities. The alarm stage signs reappear, but they are now much more difficult to reverse.

7. ANS—D *PEC—113*

An acute stress reaction may begin at the scene or shortly after the incident. The signs and symptoms may be physical, emotional, behavioral, or cognitive. They may require immediate medical attention or subsequent psychological counselling. Often, a Critical Incident Stress Debriefing process may be necessary.

8. ANS—D *PEC—114*

Delayed stress reaction, also known as post traumatic stress disorder, may appear months or years following an event. The signs and symptoms may be physical, emotional, behavioral, or cognitive. This disorder may severely affect the victim's life (i.e., marital problems, substance abuse, personality changes, suicide).

9. ANS—B *PEC—116*

Burnout occurs when coping mechanisms no longer buffer the stressors of the job. It often compromises not only the paramedic's personal health and well being, but also patient care. It is avoidable and can be prevented with early recognition and intervention.

10. ANS—D *PEC—116*

Anxiety is an emotional state caused by stress. It is characterized by increase in sympathetic nervous system tone.

11. ANS—D *PEC—118*

A certain amount of stress produces top performance and helps us cope with unusual stressors. The body has the ability to adapt to stress. The ability of the paramedic to cope with stress is often the difference between a long or short career.

12. ANS—C *PEC—117*

Many of the physiological reactions to stress are mediated by the sympathetic nervous system. Stress triggers an increase in sympathetic tone by releasing norepinephrine and epinephrine. Examples of signs and symptoms are heart palpatations, GI distress, and chest pain.

13. ANS—A *PEC—117*

Examples of physiological affects of stress include decreased circulation to the skin, increased blood pressure, increase blood glucose levels, and pupil dilation.

14. ANS—D *PEC—118*

Stress can be managed in a variety of ways. Soliciting support from co-workers, getting adequate rest and sleep, and becoming involved in things outside of EMS are some excellent ways the paramedic can begin to manage paramedic job stress.

15. ANS—D *PEC—119*

Critical Incident Stress Debriefings are structured group meetings that allow emergency and rescue personnel to openly discuss their feelings and other reactions after a critical incident. They are not psychotherapy or psychological treatments.

16. ANS—D *PEC—120*

During the acceptance stage, dying patients are without fear and despair. They are often devoid of feelings as they prepare to face death alone.

17. ANS—C *PEC—121*

When informing someone of the death of a loved one, the paramedic should use the word "dead." Avoid euphemisms such as expired, passed away, or moved on. Recognize that the family will cope with death in much the same manner as they deal with everyday stressors.

18. ANS—D *PEC—120*

During the anger stage people may project their anger at anything or anyone. This anger has little to do with the people or things present; they are simply available targets. The paramedic should allow the family to express their true feelings and not take their remarks personally. The family of the deceased now becomes the patient.

19. ANS—A *PEC—121*

The dying patient who worries about who will make the funeral arrangements is an example of reactive depression. This patient is reacting to the needs of a life situation.

20. ANS—D *PEC—121*

Stress is part of the EMS world. Paramedics must learn to deal with stress effectively and understand that too much stress can be physically and psychologically damaging.

DIVISION 2—PREPARATORY

CHAPTER 8

Medical Terminology

QUESTIONS

Give the plain English meaning for the following medical terms:

1. Adenopathy _____
2. Neuralgia _____
3. Angioplasty _____
4. Arthritis _____
5. Myasthenia _____
6. Bronchitis _____
7. Bursitis _____
8. Myocardial _____
9. Pericardiocentesis _____
10. Costochondritis _____
11. Intradermal _____
12. Abduction _____
13. Gastroenterology _____
14. Erythrocyte _____

15. Anesthesia _____
16. Afebrile _____
17. Hematuria _____
18. Hydrocephalic _____
19. Hysterectomy _____
20. Idioventricular _____
21. Nephrology _____
22. Intraosseous _____
23. Polyphagia _____
24. Pneuonectomy _____
25. Rhinorrhea _____
26. Arteriosclerosis _____
27. Hemostasis _____
28. Tachypnea _____
29. Adduction _____
30. Antihistamine _____
31. Bilateral _____
32. Bradycardia _____
33. Cerebrospinal _____
34. Contralateral _____
35. Dyspnea _____
36. Endocardium _____
37. Epidermis _____
38. Eupnea _____
39. Extrasystole _____
40. Hematoma _____
41. Hemiplegia _____
42. Hypoglycemia _____
43. Intravascular _____
44. Isotonic _____
45. Leukocyte _____
46. Oliguria _____
47. Periorbital _____
48. Arthroscopy _____
49. Retroperitoneum _____
50. Vasopressor _____

51. Sublingual   _____

52. Supraclavicular   _____

53. Transtracheal   _____

54. Unilateral   _____

55. Tracheostomy   _____

56. Laryngoscopy   _____

57. Psychosis   _____

58. Aphasia   _____

59. Photophobic   _____

60. Dysrhythmia   _____

61. Hypertrophy   _____

62. Polyuria   _____

63. Pylonephritis   _____

64. Postpartum   _____

65. Rhinoplasty   _____

Write the common abbreviations for the following terms:

66. Before   _____

67. Atherosclerotic heart disease   _____

68. Against medical advice _____

69. Blood sugar   _____

70. Body surface area   _____

71. Bag-valve-mask   _____

72. With   _____

73. Cubic centimeter   _____

74. Chief complaint   _____

75. Centimeter   _____

76. Congestive heart failure _____

77. Complains of   _____

78. Carbon monoxide   _____

79. Carbon dioxide   _____

80. Chronic obstructive pulmonary disease _____

81. Chest pain   _____

82. Cerebrospinal fluid   _____

83. Carotid sinus massage _____

84. Cerebrovasacular accident _____

85. Discontinue _____

86. Dyspnea on exertion _____

87. Deep vein thrombosis _____

88. Estimated date of confinement_____

89. Alcohol (ethanol) _____

90. Fracture _____

91. Gastrointestinal _____

92. Gunshot wound _____

93. Hour _____

94. Headache _____

95. History _____

96. Intramuscular _____

97. Intraosseous _____

98. Jugular venous distension_____

99. Potassium _____

100. Kilogram _____

101. Keep vein open _____

102. Laceration _____

103. Lactated Ringer's _____

104. Moves all extremities well_____

105. Microgram _____

106. Milliequivalent _____

107. Milligram _____

108. Milliliter _____

109. Morphine sulfate _____

110. Sodium _____

111. Sodium chloride _____

112. No known allergies _____

113. Nitroglycerine _____

114. Nausea / vomiting _____

115. Organic brain syndrome_____

116. After _____

117. Hydrogen ion concentration _____

118. Pelvic inflammatory disease _____

119. As needed _____

120. Patient _____

121. Every _____

122. Rule out _____

123. Range of motion _____

124. Without _____

125. Signs/symptoms _____

126. Subcutaneous _____

127. Sublingual _____

128. Within normal limits _____

129. Change _____

130. Year old _____

Translate the following medical report into everyday English:

Pt. is a 45 y.o. male, AO x 4, c/o sudden onset CP and SOB x 2h. Pt. also c/o DOE, N/V, and weakness. Pt. has Hx of ASHD and AMI x2 with CHF, and TIA x 1. He takes NTG 0.4mg. SL PRN for CP. NKA. VS as follows: BP 170/80, pulse 80, respirations 28, BS clear bilaterally, skin WNL. ECG shows NSR with PVC's, BS is 120. R/O AMI. Plan - O_2 - 10 LPM, NTG 0.4 mg. SL q5 minutes PRN, MS 2 mg IV repeat PRN.

ANSWERS

1. Disease of the glands

2. Pain along a nerve

3. Blood vessel repair

4. Inflammation of a joint

5. Muscle weakness

6. Inflammation of the bronchioles

7. Inflammation of the bursa

8. Pertaining to the heart muscle

9. Puncturing and draining the pericardium

10. Inflammation of the rib cartilage

11. Within the layers of the skin

12. Movement away from the body

13. The study of the GI tract

14. Red blood cell

15. Without feeling

16. Without fever

17. Blood in the urine

18. Excess water in the brain

19. Surgical removal of the uterus

20. Originating in the ventricles

21. The study of the kidneys

22. Within the bone

23. Excessive eating

24. Surgical removal of a lung

25. Runny nose

26. Hardening of the arteries

27. Standing blood

28. Rapid breathing

29. Movement toward the body

30. Against histamine (blocker)

31. On both sides

32. Slow heart (rate)

33. The brain and spine

34. On the opposite side

35. Difficulty in breathing

36. The inner heart (lining)

37. The outer skin (layer)

38. Normal breathing

39. Extra contraction (beat)

40. A blood tumor (pocket)

41. One-sided paralysis

42. Low blood sugar

43. Within a blood vessel

44. The same tone (concentration)

45. White blood cell

46. Little urine (production)

47. Around the eye orbit

48. Looking into a joint

49. Behind the peritoneum

50. An agent that constricts a blood vessel

51. Under the tongue

52. Above the clavicles

53. Across the trachea

54. On one side

55. A surgical opening into the trachea

56. Looking into the larynx

57. A mental disorder

58. Inability to speak

59. Fear of light

60. Disorganized rhythm (cardiac)

61. Overnourishment (enlargement)

62. Frequent urination

63. Kidney infection

64. After birth bleeding

65. Repair of the nose (plastic surgery)

Write the common abbreviations for the following terms:

66. $\bar{a}$

67. ASHD

68. AMA

69. BS

70. BSA

71. BVM

72. $\bar{c}$

73. cc

74. CC

75. CM

76. CHF

77. c/o

78. CO

79. CO_2

80. COPD

81. CP

82. CSF

83. CSM

84. CVA

85. D/C

86. DOE

87. DVT

88. EDC

89. ETOH

90. Fx

91. GI

92. GSW

93. h

94. H/A

95. Hx

96. IM

97. IO

98. JVD

99. K^+

100. Kg

101. KVO

102. LAC

103. LR

104. MAEW

105. Mcg

106. mEq

107. Mg

108. Ml

109. MS

110. Na$^+$

111. NaCl

112. NKA

113. NTG

114. N/V

115. OBS

116. $\bar{p}$

117. pH

118. PID

119. PRN

120. Pt

121. q

122. R/O

123. ROM

124. $\bar{s}$

125. S/S

126. SC

127. SL

128. WNL

129. Δ

130. y.o.

The patient is a 45-year-old male, alert and oriented to person, place, and time, who complains of a sudden onset of chest pain and shortness of breath that began two hours ago. The patient also complains of dyspnea upon exertion, nausea, vomiting, and weakness. The patient has a history of atherosclerotic heart disease and has had two heart attacks with congestive heart failure, and one transient ischemic attack. He takes nitroglycerine 0.4 milligrams sublingually as needed for chest pain. He has no known allergies. His vital signs are as follows: Blood pressure 170/80, pulse 80, respirations 28, breath sounds clear bilaterally, skin within normal limits. His electrocardiogram shows normal sinus rhythm with premature ventricular contractions. Blood sugar is 120. Rule out acute myocardial infarction. Plan—oxygen at 10 liters per minute; nitroglycerine 0.4 milligrams sublingually every 5 minutes as needed; Morphine sulfate 2 milligrams intravenously, repeat as needed.

CHAPTER 9

Anatomy and Physiology

QUESTIONS

1. The study of body structure is called
  A. anatomy
  B. physiology
  C. biochemistry
  D. biophysics

2. The study of body functions is called
  A. anatomy
  B. physiology
  C. biochemistry
  D. biophysics

3. The basic unit of life is the
  A. nucleus
  B. tissue
  C. organ
  D. cell

4. The organelle responsible for providing cellular energy is the
  A. nucleus
  B. mitochondria
  C. cytoplasm
  D. membrane

5. The structure that surrounds and protects the cell from the outer environment is the
   A. membrane
   B. wall
   C. mitochondria
   D. cytoplasm

6. The skin, mucous membranes, and intestinal tract lining are examples of
   A. muscle tissue
   B. connective tissue
   C. nerve tissue
   D. epithelial tissue

7. The only muscle tissue that can contract without external stimulation is
   A. cardiac muscle
   B. smooth muscle
   C. skeletal muscle
   D. connective muscle

8. Bones, cartilage, and fat are examples of
   A. epithelium
   B. organelles
   C. connective tissue
   D. organ systems

9. The type of muscle found in the inner lining of hollow organs is
   A. skeletal
   B. epithelial
   C. smooth
   D. connective

10. The natural tendency of the body to maintain a constant, stable, internal environment is called
   A. osmosis
   B. organism stability
   C. hemostasis
   D. homeostasis

11. The directional term that means "toward the midline of the body" is
   A. anterior
   B. ventral
   C. medial
   D. internal

12. The directional term that means "toward the tail" is
   A. cephalad
   B. caudad
   C. craniad
   D. dorsal

13. The distal femur is
   A. near the pelvis

    B. near the knee
    C. midshaft
    D. none of the above

14. The proximal radius articulates with the
    A. knee
    B. ankle
    C. wrist
    D. humerus

15. If the esophagus lies posterior to the trachea, it is found
    A. in front of it
    B. behind it
    C. on top of it
    D. below it

16. Lying face up is called
    A. prone
    B. Fowler's position
    C. supine
    D. Trendelenberg position

17. Elevating the head of the stretcher more than 45° is called
    A. Trendelenberg position
    B. Semi-Fowler's position
    C. Fowler's position
    D. lithotomy position

18. If your patient presents face down, he is
    A. prone
    B. supine
    C. lithotomized
    D. in Fowler's position

19. The act of moving the arm away from the body is called
    A. pronation
    B. supination
    C. abduction
    D. adduction

20. The act of rotating the arm so that the palms are face-up is called
    A. pronation
    B. supination
    C. abduction
    D. adduction

21. The act of straightening a joint is called
    A. flexion
    B. extension
    C. pronation
    D. abduction

22. The imaginary line that separates the anterior from the posterior chest is the

    A. midline
    B. mid-clavicular line
    C. mid-scapular line
    D. mid-axillary line

23. The imaginary line that extends from the manubrium to the xiphoid process is the
    A. midline
    B. mid-clavicular line
    C. mid-scapular line
    D. mid-axillary line

24. The third intercostal space is found
    A. between the 2nd and 3rd ribs
    B. between the 3rd and 4th ribs
    C. over the 3rd rib
    D. below the 4th rib

25. The lateral aspect of the abdomen is called the
    A. retroperitoneal area
    B. flank
    C. axilla
    D. pelvis

ANSWERS

1. ANS—A   *PEC—142*

Anatomy is the study of body structure.

2. ANS—B   *PEC—142*

Physiology is the study of body function.

3. ANS—D   *PEC—143*

The basic unit of life is the cell. It contains all the necessary components to turn essential nutrients into energy and to carry on essential life functions.

4. ANS—B   *PEC—144*

The mitochondria are the energy factories of the cell. They convert essential nutrients into energy sources often in the form of ATP.

5. ANS—A   *PEC—144*

The cell membrane is a structure that encircles the cell and protects it from the outer environment. It plays a major role in maintaining the internal environment of the cell.

6. ANS—D   *PEC—144*

Epithelial tissue lines body surfaces and protects the body. Certain types of epithelial tissue performs specialized functions such as secretion, absorption, diffusion, and filtration.

7. ANS—A   *PEC—144*

Cardiac muscle tissue is found only within the heart. It has the unique capability of spontaneous contraction without external stimulation. This property is called automaticity.

8. ANS—C   *PEC—144*

Connective tissue is the most abundant tissue in the body. It provides support, connection, and insulation.

9. ANS—C   *PEC—144*

The type of muscle found in the inner lining of hollow organs such as the intestines, the airways, and blood vessles is called smooth muscle. It is generally under the control of involuntary or autonomic component of the central nervous system.

10. ANS—D   *PEC—146*

The natural tendency of the body to maintain a constant, stable, internal environment is called homeostasis. The paramedic should understand this process in order to recognize how the body attempts to correct underlying problems.

11. ANS—C   *PEC—159*

The directional term that means toward the midline of the body is called medial.

12. ANS—B   *PEC—159*

The directional term that means toward the tail is called caudad.

13. ANS—B   *PEC—159*

Distal means a position further from the trunk of the body compared to another point. The distal femur is found near the knee. The proximal femur is found near the pelvis.

14. ANS—D   *PEC—159*

Proximal means near the trunk of the body compared to another point. The proximal radius articulates with the humerus.

15. ANS—B   *PEC—159*

If the esophagus lies posterior to the trachea, it is found behind it.

16. ANS—C   *PEC—159*

Lying face up is called supine.

17. ANS—C   *PEC—159*

Elevating the head of a stretcher more than 45° is called Fowler's position.

18. ANS—A   *PEC—159*

If your patient presents face down, he is prone.

19. ANS—C   *PEC—159*

The act of moving the arm away from the body is called abduction.

20. ANS—B   *PEC—159*

The act of rotating the arm so that the palms are face up is called supination.

21. ANS—B   *PEC—159*

The act of straightening a joint is called extension.

22. ANS—D   *PEC—160*

The imaginary line that separates the anterior from the posterior chest is the mid-axillary line.

23. ANS—A   *PEC—160*

The imaginary line that extends from the manubrium to the xyphoid process is the midline.

24. ANS—B   *PEC—160*

The third intercostal space is found between the third and fourth ribs.

25. ANS—B   *PEC—161*

The lateral aspect of the abdomen is called the flank.

CHAPTER 10

Advanced Patient Assessment

QUESTIONS

1. Paradoxical chest wall movement would indicate
   A. flail chest
   B. hemothorax
   C. pneumothorax
   D. traumatic asphyxia

2. In the healthy adult at rest, normal respiration should occur at a rate of
   _____ per minute.
   A. 16-22
   B. 12-20
   C. 24
   D. 60-100

3. The healthy adult at rest breathes in approximately _____ ml of air.
   A. 500
   B. 150
   C. 800
   D. 350

4. Exaggerated abdominal movement during breathing may indicate
   A. spinal cord injury
   B. diaphragmatic breathing
   C. intercostal muscle paralysis
   D. all of the above

5. The presence of supraclavicular retractions suggests
    A. hypovolemic shock
    B. decreased blood volume
    C. a partial airway obstruction
    D. cardiac arrhythmias

6. The most common cause of snoring is upper airway obstruction from
    A. foreign bodies
    B. stomach contents
    C. the tongue
    D. a swollen epiglottis

7. Snoring is best corrected by
    A. vigorous suctioning
    B. repositioning the head
    C. pumping the stomach
    D. endotracheal intubation

8. High pitched "crowing" sounds caused by obstruction of the upper airway are called
    A. wheezes
    B. snoring
    C. rales
    D. stridor

9. The whistling sounds indicative of lower airway constriction are called
    A. wheezes
    B. snoring
    C. rales
    D. stridor

10. Your patient presents unconscious, without a gag reflex, and moving less than 6 liters/minute of air. You should do all of the following **EXCEPT**
    A. Intubate the patient
    B. Perform bag-valve-mask ventilations
    C. Administer 100% oxygen
    D. Complete the primary survey before treating

11. Your patient presents with warm, pink skin, radial pulse rate of 80/minute, and capillary refill time of :02 seconds. From this information what can you conclude about her circulatory condition?
    A. It is normal
    B. It shows signs of early circulatory compromise
    C. It shows signs of severe circulatory collapse
    D. None of the above

12. Which of the following is **NOT** a physical exam technique?
    A. Palpitation
    B. Auscultation
    C. Percussion
    D. Inspection

13. Heart sounds can best be heard by placing the stethoscope over the

    A. apex of the heart
    B. fourth intercostal space, right mid-clavicular line
    C. third intercostal space, just left of the sternum
    D. fifth intercostal space, mid-axillary line

14. A hollow and vibrating resonance heard when percussing the chest indicates the presence of
    A. air
    B. blood
    C. pleural fluid
    D. water

15. A black-and-bluish discoloration over the mastoid process is called
    A. periorbital ecchymosis
    B. Battle's sign
    C. raccoon's eyes
    D. Cushing's reflex

16. A positive halo test indicates the presence of
    A. sugar
    B. blood
    C. stomach contents
    D. cerebrospinal fluid

17. Pinpoint pupils indicate
    A. severe brain injury
    B. hypoxia
    C. intracranial pressure
    D. opiate overdose

18. Failure of the eyes to rotate simultaneously in the same direction is called
    A. anisocoria
    B. dysconjugate gaze
    C. doll'e eye reflex
    D. Battle's sign

Match the following oral cavity fluids with their possible pathologies:

19.	_____	Coffee grounds	**A.**	Congestive heart failure
20.	_____	Fresh blood	**B.**	Respiratory infection
21.	_____	Pink-tinged sputum	**C.**	Bleeding in the stomach
22.	_____	Green or yellow phlegm	**D.**	Brainstem problem
23.	_____	Vomit	**E.**	Upper GI hemorrhage

24. Significant jugular venous distension is evaluated with the patient's body at a _____ angle.
    A. 90°
    B. 45°
    C. 0°
    D. 180°

25. Significant JVD is indicative of

   A. hypovolemia
   B. hypotension
   C. cardiac tamponade
   D. left heart failure

26. Your patient is lying supine and his neck veins are flat. You conclude that he
   A. has a tension pneumothorax
   B. has right heart failure
   C. is hypovolemic
   D. has cor pulmonale

27. The presence of air just underneath the surface of the skin is known as
   A. pulmonary emphysema
   B. subcutaneous emphysema
   C. crepital emphysema
   D. ipsilateral emphysema

28. A rapid, deep respiratory pattern may be indicative of
   A. a head injury
   B. extreme exertion
   C. a diabetic problem
   D. all of the above

29. A series of increasing, then decreasing, breaths with periods of apnea in between is known as
   A. Biot's
   B. Kussmaul's
   C. Central neurogenic hyperventilation
   D. Cheyne-Stokes

30. A bluish discoloration around the umbilicus is known as
   A. Grey-Turner's sign
   B. Cullen's sign
   C. Cushing's reflex
   D. Battle's sign

31. Rebound tenderness is indicative of
   A. peritoneal inflammation
   B. impending aortic aneurysm rupture
   C. solid organ inflammation
   D. none of the above

32. Ascites is caused by
   A. increased portal circulation
   B. right heart failure
   C. cirrhosis of the liver
   D. all of the above

33. Presacral edema is indicative of
   A. congestive heart failure
   B. peritoneal irritation
   C. cirrhosis of the liver

D. ruptured ipsilateral kidney

34. Priapism is caused by
A. unopposed parasympathetic stimulation
B. spinal cord interruption
C. brain dysfunction
D. all of the above

35. Clubbing is caused by
A. a chronic hypoxic condition
B. cardiovascular and pulmonary disease
C. central cyanosis
D. all of the above

36. The difference between systolic and diastolic blood pressures is known as
A. pulsus paradoxus
B. mean arterial pressure
C. central venous pressure
D. pulse pressure

37. If your supine patient's pulse rate rises more than 15 beats per minute when you sit him up, what should you suspect?
A. congestive heart failure
B. significant blood loss
C. severe hypertension
D. coronary artery disease

38. Patients with effective respiration should measure an oxygen saturation of
A. 80—100 mg/kg
B. 120 d/L
C. 90—100 torr
D. 96—100%

39. In which of the following situations might your oximetry reading be misleading?
A. Severe hypothermia
B. Carbon monoxide poisoning
C. Hypovolemia
D. All of the above

40. The primary sign or symptom noticed by the patient is called the
A. primary problem
B. associated symptom
C. chief complaint
D. history of present illness

41. When recording your patient's symptoms, it is best to use
A. medical terminology
B. the patient's own words
C. your interpretation
D. none of the above

42. Often the pain of myocardial infarction is felt in the neck and jaw. This is known as _____ pain.
A. aggravating
B. alleviating
C. radiating
D. referred

43. The "P" in the mnemonic "AMPLE" stands for
A. palleative factors
B. provocative factors
C. past medical history
D. personal physician

44. The "M" in the mnemonic "AMPLE" stands for
A. medications
B. medical history
C. monitor
D. movement

45. The "A" in the mnemonic "AMPLE" stands for
A. allergies
B. attacks
C. aggravating factors
D. alleviating factors

ANSWERS   **1. ANS—A**   *PEC—171*

Paradoxical movement of the chest wall is when the chest wall moves in a fashion opposite to that expected. It's often seen in flail chest injuries where the flail segment moves in an opposite direction compared to the rest of the chest. This is caused by changes in pressures within the chest wall.

2. ANS—B   *PEC—172*

In the healthy adult at rest normal respirations should occur at a rate of 12-20 breaths per minute.

3. ANS—A   *PEC—172*

A healthy adult at rest breathes in approximately 500 ml of air. This is known as tidal volume.

4. ANS—D   *PEC—172*

Exaggerated abdominal movement during breathing may indicate that the diaphram is the only muscle being used. It may be a result of spinal cord injury or intercostal muscle paralysis in which the other muscles of breathing are no longer functional.

5. ANS—C   *PEC—172*

Retraction means the act of drawing back or inward. In the case of partial airway obstruction an increased inspiratory effort causes great pressures within the chest wall. These pressures cause the tissue between the ribs and sternal notch to retract or move inward.

6. ANS—C   *PEC—172*

The most common cause of snoring is upper airway obstruction from the tongue. This is generally caused by gravity moving the relaxed tongue into the posterior pharnyx. In the unconscious person this is to be expected.

7. ANS—B   *PEC—172*

Snoring is best corrected by repositioning the head. If you do not suspect your patient having a cervical spine injury, use the head-tilt chin lift method. In the trauma patient, when cervical spine integrity is compromised, use the modified jaw thrust.

8. ANS—D   *PEC—172*

High pitched "crowing sounds" caused by obstruction of the upper airway are called stridor. These sounds indicate severe obstruction in the upper airway and are very difficult to correct in the field. Suspect a foreign body or tissue swelling phenomenon.

9. ANS—A   *PEC—172*

The whistling sounds indicative of lower airway obstruction are called wheezes. These are whistling type breath sounds associated with narrowing or spasm of the smaller airways.

10. ANS—D   *PEC—172*

If your patient presents unconscious without a gag reflex and moving less than six liters per minute of air, you should first perform bag-valve mask ventilations with 100% oxygen and plan to intubate the patient.

11. ANS—A   *PEC—172*

Normal circulatory status is evidenced by warm, dry skin, the presence of a radial pulse at a rate of 60-100 per minute, and capillary refill time of less than two seconds.

12. ANS—A   *PEC—177*

Four common physical exam techniques are inspection, palpation, ausculation, and percussion.

13. ANS—C   *PEC—177*

You may choose to evaluate heart sounds by ausculation. Use the bell side of your stethoscope to pick up the closing of the valves and any extraneous sounds. Place the bell lightly over the heart valves at approximately the third intercostal space just left of the sternum.

14. ANS—A   *PEC—178*

Percussion evaluates the surface and the tissue beneath by sending a vibration through it. A hollow and vibrating residence heard when percussing the chest indicates the presence of air.

15. ANS—B   *PEC—179*

Battle's sign is a black and blue discoloration over the mastoid process just behind the ear. This is characteristic of a basilar skull fracture. It is not commonly seen in the prehospital setting because it takes several hours to produce the discoloration.

16. ANS—D *PEC—179*

The halo test is performed by dropping the fluid in question onto a gauze pad or a sheet. If blood and cerebral spinal fluid are mixed, it will yield a characteristic halo or target sign (darker red circles surrounded by a lighter one). This indicates the presence of cerebrospinal spinal fluid in the blood.

17. ANS—D *PEC—180*

Very small or pin-point pupils suggest intoxication from opium derivatives (narcotics, heroin, morphine, percodan, darvon, codeine).

18. ANS—B *PEC—180*

Failure of the eyes to rotate simultaneously in the same direction is called dysconjugate gaze. This may indicate a pre-existing problem, occular muscle intrapment, or optic nerve damage. Do not attempt this maneuver on any patient with suspected spine injury.

19. _____	Coffee grounds	C.	Bleeding in the stomach	*PEC—181*
20. _____	Fresh blood	E.	Upper GI hemorrhage	
21. _____	Pink-tinged sputum	A.	Congestive heart failure	
22. _____	Green or yellow phlegm	B.	Respiratory infection	
23. _____	Vomit	D.	Brainstem problem	

24. ANS—B *PEC—182*

You should always examine the jugular veins for distention. In the supine normotensive patient, they should distend slightly. However, as the body is brought to a 45° angle they empty. Distention beyond 45° is indicative of pathology.

25. ANS—C *PEC—182*

Significant jugular venous distention is indicative of cardiac tamponade, tension pneumothorax, right heart failure, or corpulmonale.

26. ANS—C *PEC—182*

If the veins do not distend in the supine position, hypovolemia is the probable cause.

27. ANS—B *PEC—183*

Subcutaneous emphysema is the presence of air within the subcutanous tissues often associated with pneumothorax. Palpating the skin in this area will produce a crackling sound and feeling.

28. ANS—D *PEC—185*

A rapid, deep respiratory pattern could be due to head injury (central neurogenic hyperventilation), a metabolic problem (diabetic coma), extreme exertion, or hyperventilation syndrome.

29. ANS—D *PEC—185*

Cheyne-Stokes is a respiratory pattern characterized by progressive increase in the rate and volume of respirations that later gradually subsides. It is usually associated with a disturbance in the respiratory center of the brain.

30. ANS—B   *PEC—186*

Cullen's sign is a bluish discoloration of the area around the umbilicus caused by intra-abdominal hemorrhage.

31. ANS—A   *PEC—186*

Rebound tenderness is a physical finding of tenderness upon sudden release of an examining hand from the abdomen often associated with peritoneal irritation.

32. ANS—D   *PEC—186*

Ascites is an accumulation of fluid within the abdominal cavity. It is often caused by increased pressure in the systemic circulation (right heart failure) or in the portal system (cirrhosis of the liver). It is associated with congestive heart failure and alcoholism among other causes.

33. ANS—A   *PEC—187*

Presacral edema is an accumulation of fluid in flank area in the recumbent patient. This is usually related to congestive heart failure.

34. ANS—D   *PEC—187*

Priapism is a painful prolonged erection of the penis. It results from unopposed parasympathetic stimulation. It occurs with spinal cord interruption or certain types of brain dysfunction.

35. ANS—B   *PEC—189*

Clubbing is an enlargement of the distal fingers and toes often due to chronic respiratory or cardiovascular disease.

36. ANS—D   *PEC—193*

The difference between systolic and diastolic blood pressures is known as pulse pressure. The patient with a blood pressure of 120/80 has a pulse pressure of 40.

37. ANS—B   *PEC—193*

If your supine patient's pulse rate rises more than 15 beats per minute when you sit him up, you should suspect a significant blood loss. This is known as a positive "tilt test," or orthostatic hypotension.

38. ANS—D   *PEC—195*

Patients with effective respirations should measure an oxygen saturation of 96-100%. If respirations are compromised even slightly, oxygen saturation falls. Provide any patient whose saturation is below 90% with aggressive oxygenation and possibly positive pressure ventilation.

39. ANS—D   *PEC—195*

Pulse oximeter measures the oxygen saturation level of blood through a non-invasive sensor placed on a finger or ear lobe. In low flow states, such as hypothermia and late hypovolemia, the device may not sense accurately. The presence of a carbon monoxide on the hemoglobin molecule tends to elevate the saturation level falsely.

40. ANS—C   *PEC—197*

The primary presenting symptom noticed by the patient is called the chief complaint. It is the reason that caused your patient to request help.

41. ANS—B *PEC—197*

When describing your patient's symptoms, it is best to use the patient's own words. In other words, your patient is "having trouble breathing," not "dyspneic."

42. ANS—D *PEC—198*

Referred pain is pain that is referred to other parts of the body. The two most common areas that produce referred pain are the heart and the diaphram. Pain from the heart is most commonly referred to the left arm. The pain associated with diapramatic irritation is generally referred to the clavical region.

43. ANS—C *PEC—200*

The P in AMPLE stands for past medical history.

44. ANS—A *PEC—200*

The M in AMPLE stands for medications taken.

45. ANS—A *PEC—200*

The A in AMPLE stands for allergies.

CHAPTER 11

Advanced Airway Management and Ventilation

QUESTIONS

1. Which of the following is a responsibility of the nasal cavity?
   A. Filter the incoming air
   B. Humidify the incoming air
   C. Warm the incoming air
   D. All of the above

2. What purpose do the conchae serve?
   A. They secrete mucus into the nasal cavity
   B. They propell foreign particles into the pharynx
   C. They cause air flow turbulence
   D. They stimulate the cilia

3. The muscular tube that extends from the back of the soft palate to the esophagus is the
   A. trachea
   B. larynx
   C. pharynx
   D. eustachian tube

4. A leaf-shaped cartilage that prevents food from entering the larynx during swallowing is the
   A. arytenoid
   B. cricoids

    C. epiglottis
    D. hyoid

5. The depression between the epiglottis and the base of the tongue is the
    A. eustachian tube
    B. vallecula
    C. hyoid
    D. pyriform fossa

6. The narrowest part of the adult upper airway is at the level of the
    A. vocal cords
    B. cricoid cartilage
    C. cricothyroid membrane
    D. hyoid bone

7. The space between the vocal cords is known as the
    A. eustachian tube
    B. hyoid process
    C. cricothyroid membrane
    D. glottis

8. The trachea divides into the right and left mainstem bronchi at the
    A. hyoid bone
    B. carina
    C. vallecula
    D. parenchyma

9. An endotracheal tube inserted too far will most likely rest in the
    A. right mainstem bronchus
    B. left mainstem bronchus
    C. lung parenchyma
    D. carina

10. Most gas exchange occurs in the
    A. respiratory bronchioles
    B. alveoli
    C. alveolar ducts
    D. bronchioles

11. The _____ pleura covers the lungs.
    A. visceral
    B. parietal
    C. pulmonary
    D. respiratory

12. During inspiration, air enters the lungs because of a/an _____ in intrathoracic pressure.
    A. increase
    B. decrease

13. The lungs receive deoxygenated blood from the
    A. right heart
    B. left heart

    C. pulmonary veins

    D. bronchial arteries

14. The normal PaO_2 for a healthy adult breathing room air is _____ torr.

    A. 60

    B. 80–100

    C. 35–45

    D. 40

15. The normal $PaCO_2$ for a healthy adult breathing room air is _____ torr.

    A. 60–80

    B. 80–100

    C. 35–45

    D. 7.35–7.45

16. Oxygen molecules move from the alveoli into the pulmonary capillary because of a process known as

    A. osmosis

    B. ventilation/perfusion mismatch

    C. atelectasis

    D. diffusion

17. 97% of the oxygen that enters the bloodstream

    A. is dissolved in plasma

    B. binds with hemoglobin

    C. is transported as bicarbonate

    D. is exhaled into the atmosphere

18. In which of the following cases would the oxygen saturation and partial pressure be high yet the patient die of hypoxia?

    A. Carbon monoxide poisoning

    B. Hypothermia

    C. Hypovolemia

    D. All of the above

19. Which of the following conditions might cause a ventilation/perfusion mismatch?

    A. Pneumothorax

    B. Hemothorax

    C. Pulmonary embolism

    D. All of the above

20. The FiO_2 of room air is

    A. 80–100 torr

    B. 21%

    C. 100 %

    D. 40 torr

21. When it enters the bloodstream, the majority of carbon dioxide

    A. is dissolved in plasma

    B. binds with hemoglobin

    C. is transported as bicarbonate

    D. combines with carbon monoxide

22. Which of the following would **NOT** increase a patient's $PaCO_2$?
    A. Hyperventilation
    B. Hypoventilation
    C. Airway obstruction
    D. Muscle exertion

23. The main respiratory center lies in the
    A. apneustic center
    B. pneumotaxic center
    C. stretch receptors
    D. medulla

24. The Hering-Breuer Reflex is a process that
    A. ensures rhythmic inspiration
    B. monitors for changes in $PaCO_2$
    C. prevents overinflation of the lungs
    D. controls hypoxic drive

25. Chemoreceptors are stimulated by which of the following
    A. increased PaO_2
    B. increased $PaCO_2$
    C. increased pH
    D. none of the above

26. Patients with hypoxic drive are stimulated to breathe by
    A. increases in PaO_2
    B. decreases in $PaCO_2$
    C. increases in pH
    D. none of the above

Match the following modified forms of respiration with their descriptions:

27. ____	Coughing	**A.**	Prolonged exhalation
28. ____	Sneezing	**B.**	Respiratory distress sign in infants
29. ____	Hiccoughing	**C.**	Protective airway function
30. ____	Sighing	**D.**	Caused by nasal irritation
31. ____	Grunting	**E.**	Diaphragmatic spasm

32. The average volume of gas inhaled in one respiratory cycle is known as
    A. minute volume
    B. tidal volume
    C. alveolar volume
    D. none of the above

33. Maximum lung capacity in the average adult male is approximately
    A. 4500 ml
    B. 350 ml
    C. 6000 ml
    D. 500 ml

34. The average tidal volume in the healthy adult male is approximately
  A. 150 ml
  B. 500 ml
  C. 350 ml
  D. 6000 ml

35. Minute volume is calculated
  A. respiratory rate × dead air space
  B. tidal volume – dead air space
  C. alveolar volume ÷ dead air space
  D. tidal volume × respiratory rate

36. The stiffness or flexibility of the lungs is known as
  A. capnography
  B. compliance
  C. saturation
  D. atelectasis

37. Upper airway obstruction can be caused by
  A. anaphylaxis
  B. epiglottitis
  C. respiratory burns
  D. all of the above

38. Sellick's maneuver is used to
  A. prevent regurgitation
  B. aid in EOA insertion
  C. open the airway in trauma
  D. all of the above

39. Your patient is semi-conscious with a gag reflex. Which of the following airway adjuncts is indicated?
  A. Oropharyngeal Airway
  B. Nasopharyngeal Airway
  C. Endotracheal tube
  D. Esophageal Obturator Airway

40. The major advantage of using a nasopharyngeal airway is that
  A. it isolates the trachea
  B. it is easy to suction through
  C. it can be used in the presence of a gag reflex
  D. none of the above

41. The distal cuff on an endotracheal tube should be filled with _____ ml of air.
  A. 5–10
  B. 10–20
  C. 20–30
  D. 30–35

42. Noncuffed endotracheal tubes are recommended for children under the age of

     A. 5 years
     B. 8 years
     C. 10 years
     D. 12 years

43. Endotracheal intubation may be attempted in all of the following situations **EXCEPT**
     A. patients without a gag reflex
     B. anaphylaxis
     C. respiratory burns
     D. epiglottitis

44. Which of the following drugs may **NOT** be administered down the endotracheal tube?
     A. Epinephrine
     B. Atropine
     C. Lidocaine
     D. Sodium Bicarbonate

45. Each endotracheal intubation attempt should be limited to _____ seconds.
     A. 10
     B. 15
     C. 30
     D. 60

46. The endotracheal tube may be misplaced into which of the following structures?
     A. Esophagus
     B. Pyriform sinus
     C. Vallecula
     D. All of the above

47. Which of the following indicates an esophageal intubation?
     A. Phonation
     B. Absence of breath sounds
     C. Gurgling sounds heard over the epigastrium
     D. All of the above

48. The proper position of the head and neck for endotracheal intubation in the non-trauma patient is the _____ position.
     A. neutral
     B. hyperextended
     C. sniffing
     D. flexed

49. The curved, or Macintosh, blade is designed to
     A. lift the epiglottitis
     B. spread the vocal cords
     C. fit into the vallecula
     D. none of the above

50. If your intubated patient has breath sounds only over the right chest, you should
   A. remove the tube immediately
   B. secure the tube in place
   C. bring the tube back a few centimeters and recheck
   D. push the tube in a few centimeters and recheck

51. Which of the following is true regarding suctioning
   A. It should be limited to 30 seconds
   B. Apply suction during insertion and during removal
   C. Hyperventilate the patient before and after suctioning
   D. All of the above

52. The nasal cannula delivers oxygen concentrations in the range of
   A. 10–50%
   B. 50–100%
   C. 24–44%
   D. 40–60%

53. Nasal cannula flow rates should not exceed _____ lpm.
   A. 3
   B. 6
   C. 8
   D. 10

54. The simple face mask delivers oxygen concentrations in the range of
   A. 20–40%
   B. 40–60%
   C. 60–80%
   D. 80–100%

55. Simple face mask flow rates should never fall below _____ lpm.
   A. 3
   B. 6
   C. 8
   D. 10

56. The nonrebreather mask delivers oxygen concentrations in the range of
   A. 20–40%
   B. 40–60%
   C. 60–80%
   D. 80–100%

57. Nonrebreather mask flow rates should never fall below _____ lpm.
   A. 3
   B. 6
   C. 8
   D. 10

58. The Venturi system delivers oxygen concentrations in the range of
   A. 24–40%
   B. 40–60%
   C. 60–80%

D. 80–100%

59. To achieve effective ventilatory support you must deliver at least _____ ml of oxygen at a rate of _____ breaths per minute.
A. 300, 16–20
B. 500, 12–22
C. 800, 12–20
D. 1000, 16–24

60. Using a pocket mask without supplemental oxygen delivers oxygen in the range of
A. 16–17%
B. 21–22 %
C. 20–50%
D. 90–100%

61. A bag-valve-mask device with an oxygen reservoir can deliver up to _____ of oxygen with flow rates at 10–15 lpm.
A. 50%
B. 60%
C. 80%
D. 95%

62. A demand valve resuscitator will deliver up to _____ oxygen at its highest flow rates.
A. 50%
B. 60%
C. 80%
D. 100%

63. Which of the following complications is associated with demand valve use?
A. pneumothorax
B. subcutaneous emphysema
C. gastric distention
D. all of the above

64. Which of the following is true regarding the use of an automatic ventilator?
A. They deliver higher minute volumes than the bag-valve-mask
B. Most units deliver controlled ventilation only
C. They can be used safely in all age groups
D. The pop-off valves should be disengaged

65. In which of the following cases might higher airway pressures be necessary to ventilate the lungs?
A. Cardiogenic pulmonary edema
B. Adult Respiratory Distress Syndrome
C. Bronchospasm
D. All of the above

ANSWERS   **1. ANS—D**   *PEC—210*

The nasal cavity is responsible for filtering, humidifying, and warming the incoming air.

2. ANS—C   *PEC—210*

The conchae or turbinates are shelf-like structures that cause turbulent airflow. This turbulence helps deposit any airborne particles onto the mucus membrane that lines the nasal cavity.

3. ANS—C   *PEC—210*

The pharynx, or throat, is a muscular tube that extends vertically from the back of the soft palate to the upper end of the esophagus. It allows the flow of air into and out of the respiratory tract and the passage of foods and liquids into the digestive system.

4. ANS—C   *PEC—210*

The epiglottis is a leaf-shaped cartilage that prevents food from entering the respiratory tract during the act of swallowing.

5. ANS—B   *PEC—210*

The depression between the epiglottis and the base of the tongue is known as the vallecula. This landmark is significant because during intubation, you insert the curved blade into this crevice.

6. ANS—A   *PEC—211*

In adults the portion of the thyroid cartilage housing the vocal cords is the narrowest part of the upper airway.

7. ANS—D   *PEC—211*

The glottis is the slit-like opening between the vocal cords, also known as the glottic opening.

8. ANS—B   *PEC—213*

The carina is the point at which the trachea bifurcates into the right and left mainstem bronchi.

9. ANS—A   *PEC—213*

The right mainstem bronchus is almost straight and slightly curved where the left main bronchus angles more acutely to the left. An endotracheal tube inserted too far will most likely rest in the right mainstem bronchus for that reason.

10. ANS—B   *PEC—213*

A limited gas exchange may occur in the alveolar ducts and respiratory bronchioles. Most gas exchange takes place in the alveoli. The alveoli comprise the key functional unit of the respiratory system.

11. ANS—A   *PEC—213*

Lungs are covered by connective tissue called pleura. The pleura consists of two layers, the visceral pleura covers the lungs and does not contain nerve fibers.

12. ANS—B   *PEC—214*

During inspiration the size of the thoracic cavity is made larger by contracting the diaphragm and the intercostal muscles. This causes a great and instant decrease in the intrathoracic pressure. This decrease in intrathoracic pressure causes air to rush into the lungs.

13. ANS—A *PEC—214*

The lungs receive deoxygenated blood from the right side of the heart through the pulmonary artery. The pulmonary artery is the only artery in the body that carries deoxygenated blood.

14. ANS—B *PEC—216*

The normal PaO_2 for a healthy adult breathing room air is 80-100 torr.

15. ANS—C *PEC—216*

The normal $PaCO_2$ for a healthy adult breathing room air is 35-45 torr.

16. ANS—D *PEC—216*

Diffusion is the movement of gas from an area of higher partial pressure concentration to an area of lower partial pressure concentration. This process allows oxygen molecules to move from the alveoli into the pulmonary capillary.

17. ANS—B *PEC—216*

Of the oxygen that enters the bloodstream, 97% of it binds with the hemoglobin molecule on the red blood cells. Three percent is dissolved in plasma.

18. ANS—A *PEC—216*

Consider the patient with carbon monoxide poisoning. Since carbon monoxide has a greater affinity for the hemoglobin molecule than oxygen does, it will replace it, if present. That means that most of the oxygen inhaled will be dissolved in plasma. If arterial blood gas samples were taken, it would reveal a normal or high PaO_2 because the PaO_2 measures the freely dissolved oxygen in the bloodstream. The pulse oximeter measures the saturation of the hemoglobin molecule. In this case, it is saturated not with oxygen but with carbon monoxide. Both measurements would read high yet the patient would die of hypoxia. It's the hemoglobin that transports oxygen to the peripheral tissues.

19. ANS—D *PEC—217*

Ideally, each milliliter of air we inhale should meet up with 1 ml of blood. When it doesn't, a ventilation/perfusion mismatch occurs. This can be caused by a problem with ventilation or a problem with circulation. Ventilation-perfusion mismatches are the most common cause of respiratory distress.

20. ANS—B *PEC—217*

The FiO_2 is a measurement of the concentration of oxygen in the inspired air. The FiO_2 of room air is approximately .21 (21%).

21. ANS—C *PEC—217*

Carbon dioxide is transported mainly in the form of bicarbonate. Approximately 66% is transported in this manner while 33% is transported combined with hemoglobin. Less than 1 percent is dissolved in the plasma.

22. ANS—A *PEC—217*

Carbon dioxide concentrations in the blood are influenced by increases and decreases in CO_2 production and/or elimination. $PaCO_2$ would be increased by hypoventilation, airway obstruction, or muscle exertion.

23. ANS—D   *PEC—218*

The respiratory center lies in the medulla located in the brain stem.

24. ANS—C   *PEC—218*

The Hering-Breuer reflex is a process that prevents over expansion of the lungs. During inspiration the lungs become distended activating what are known as stretch receptors. As the degree of stretch increases, these receptors fire more frequently sending a message to the brain stem to inhibit the respiratory inspiration.

25. ANS—B   *PEC—218*

Receptors are located in the carotid bodies, the aortic arch, and in the medulla. In the normal person these chemoreceptors are stimulated by decreased PaO_2, increased $PaCO_2$, and a decreased pH.

26. ANS—D   *PEC—218*

People with chronic respiratory disease such as emphysema and chronic bronchitis tend to retain carbon dioxide and often develop a condition known as hypoxic drive. These patients are stimulated to breath by decreases in PaO_2.

27. _____	Coughing	**C.** Protective airway function	*PEC—219*
28. _____	Sneezing	**D.** Caused by nasal irritation	
29. _____	Hiccoughing	**E.** Diaphragmatic spasm	
30. _____	Sighing	**A.** Prolonged exhalation	
31. _____	Grunting	**B.** Respiratory distress sign in infants	

32. ANS—B   *PEC—219*

Tidal volume is the average volume of gas inhaled or exhaled in one respiratory cycle.

33. ANS—C   *PEC—219*

Total lung capacity in the average adult male is approximately six liters.

34. ANS—B   *PEC—219*

The average tidal volume in a healthy adult male is approximately 500 ml.

35. ANS—D   *PEC—220*

Minute volume is the amount of gas moved in and out of the respiratory tract in one minute. It is measured by multiplying the tidal volume times the respiratory rate.

36. ANS—B   *PEC—224*

Compliance refers to the stiffness or flexibility to the lung tissue. It is determined by how easily air flows into the lungs. When compliance is good, airflow occurs with a minimal amount of resistance. Poor compliance means that ventilation is harder to achieve. It is often poor in diseased lungs, patients with chest wall injuries, or tension pneumothorax.

37. ANS—D   *PEC—226*

Upper airway obstruction can be caused by anaphylaxis, epiglottitis, and respiratory burns.

38. ANS—A *PEC—230*

Sellick's maneuver is used to prevent regurgitation by applying slight pressure posteriorly over the cricoid cartilage thus closing off the esophagus. It is also useful in endotracheal intubation to help bring the larynx into view.

39. ANS—B *PEC—233*

In the semi-conscious patient with a gag reflex, the nasopharyngeal airway is an excellent initial airway adjunct.

40. ANS—C *PEC—233*

The major advantage of using the nasopharyngeal airway is that it can be used in the presence of the gag reflex.

41. ANS—A *PEC—242*

The cuff of an endotracheal tube should be filled with 5-10 ml of air.

42. ANS—B *PEC—242*

Non-cuffed endotracheal tubes are recommended for children under the age of 8-years-old. In these children the cricoid cartilage acts as an anatomical cuff since it is the narrowest part of the pediatric airway.

43. ANS—D *PEC—243*

Tracheal intubation should never be attempted in patients suspected of having epiglottis. Any unecessary agitation of the patient can cause immediate laryngospasm and subsequent respiratory arrest.

44. ANS—D *PEC—243*

The following medications can be administered down the endotracheal tube: oxygen, naloxone, atropine, diazepam, epinephrine, lidocaine.

45. ANS—C *PEC—244*

According to the American Heart Association, endotracheal intubation attempts should be limited to no more than 30 seconds to prevent hypoxia.

46. ANS—D *PEC—245*

The endotracheal tube may be misplaced into the esophagus, the pyriform sinus, or the vallecula.

47. ANS—D *PEC—245*

Signs of an esophageal intubation include an absence of chest rise and breath sounds with ventilatory support; gurgling sounds heard over the epigastrium; the absence of breath condensation in the endotracheal tube; a persistent air leak despite inflation of the distal cuff; cyanosis; progressive worsening of the patient's condition, and phonation.

48. ANS—C *PEC—245*

The proper position of the head and neck for endotracheal intubation in the non-trauma patient is the sniffing position. This is accomplished by flexing the neck forward and the head backward or by inserting a roll towel under the patient's shoulders or the back of the head.

49. ANS—C *PEC—245*

The curved, or Macintosh, blade is designed to fit into the vallecula. The vallecula is the space between the base of the tongue and the epiglottis.

50. ANS—C *PEC—248*

If your intubated patient has breath sounds heard only over the right chest, you should assume a right mainstem bronchus intubation. In this case, withdraw the tube back a few centimeters and recheck placement.

51. ANS—C *PEC—277*

Suctioning should always be limited to 15 seconds. You should hyperventilate the patient before and after all suctioning attempts and always apply suction during removal.

52. ANS—C *PEC—279*

The nasal cannula delivers oxygen concentrations in the range of 24–44% depending on the liter flow.

Nasal Cannula Oxygen Delivery	
Liter Flow	**Approximate Oxygen Concentration Delivered**
1	24
2	28
3	32
4	36
5	40
6	44

53. ANS—B *PEC—280*

Nasal cannulla flow rates should not exceed 6 liters per minute as this will dry the mucus membrane and cause headaches.

54. ANS—B *PEC—281*

The simple face mask delivers oxygen concentrations in the range of 40-60%. Oxygen is delivered through the bottom of the mask via its oxygen inlet port.

55. ANS—B *PEC—281*

No fewer than 6 liters per minute should be administered through this device as expired carbon dioxide can otherwise accumulate in the mask.

56. ANS—D *PEC—281*

The nonrebreather mask consists of oxygen tubing and a face mask with an attached reservoir bag. When the patient inhales, 100% oxygen contained in the reservoir is drawn into the mask and the patient's respiratory passageways. The nonrebreather mask delivers the highest concentration of oxygen. Once applied a flowrate of 10-15 liters per minute can deliver an 80-100% oxygen concentration.

57. ANS—C *PEC—281*

No fewer than 8 liters of oxygen per minute should be administered through this device.

58. ANS—A *PEC—282*

The venturi system is a high flow device including oxygen tubing, a face mask, and the venturi system. As oxygen passes through a jet port in the base of the mask, it entrains room air. Depending on the device used, oxygen concentrations can be delivered in the range of 24-40%.

59. ANS—C   *PEC—283*

To achieve adequate ventilatory support, you must deliver at least 800 ml of oxygen at a rate of 12-20 breaths per minute.

60. ANS—A   *PEC—283*

Using a pocket mask without supplemental oxygen delivers the oxygen in the range of 16-17%. In other words your own expired FiO_2.

61. ANS—D   *PEC—284*

A bag-valve mask device with an oxygen reservoir can deliver up to 95% of oxygen with flow rates at 10-15 liters per minute.

62. ANS—D   *PEC—284*

A demand valve resuscitator will deliver up to 100% oxygen at its highest flow rates.

63. ANS—D   *PEC—284*

Using a demand valve has its disadvantages. Some of these include creating a pneumothorax, subcutaneous emphysema, or gastric distension.

64. ANS—A   *PEC—286*

Automatic ventilators deliver higher minute volumes than the bag-valve mask.

65. ANS—D   *PEC—286*

In cases such as cardiodemic pulmonary edema, adult respiratory distress syndrome, and bronchospasm, higher airway pressures may be necessary to ventilate the lungs.

CHAPTER 12

Pathophysiology of Shock

QUESTIONS

1. Water makes up approximately _____ of total body weight.
   A. 30%
   B. 60%
   C. 80%
   D. none of the above

2. Where is most of this water is found?
   A. Between the cells
   B. In the blood vessels
   C. In the cells
   D. None of the above

3. All of the following happens when your fluid levels drop EXCEPT
   A. ADH is secreted
   B. the kidneys reabsorb sodium
   C. more urine is excreted
   D. water shifts into the intravascular compartment

4. All of the following are signs of dehydration EXCEPT
   A. poor skin turgor
   B. sacral edema
   C. sunken fontanelles
   D. tachycardia

5. Dehydrated patients should receive
    A. an isotonic solution
    B. Lactated Ringer's
    C. normal saline
    D. all of the above

6. A medication that stimulates the kidneys to excrete water is a/an
    A. cation
    B. anion
    C. diuretic
    D. homeostatic

7. A positively charged ion is called a/an
    A. cation
    B. anion
    C. colloid
    D. crystalloid

8. The chief extracellular cation that regulates fluid distribution is
    A. bicarbonate
    B. sodium
    C. potassium
    D. magnesium

9. The chief intracellular cation that aids in electrical impulse transmission is
    A. magnesium
    B. sodium
    C. potassium
    D. calcium

10. The cation that plays a major role in muscle contraction is
    A. bicarbonate
    B. sodium
    C. potassium
    D. calcium

11. The principle buffer of the acid-base system is
    A. bicarbonate
    B. sodium
    C. potassium
    D. magnesium

12. Electrolytes are measured in
    A. mg/kg
    B. mEq/L
    C. mEq/dl
    D. mcg/L

13. The movement of water through a semi-permeable membrane from an area of low solute concentration toward an area of high solute concentration is called
    A. diffusion

    B. facilitated diffusion
    C. active transport
    D. osmosis

14. Infusing a hypotonic solution into the bloodstream will cause water to move in the following direction:
    A. into the cells
    B. into the bloodvessel
    C. out of the cells
    D. none of the above

15. The movement of solute particles through a semi-permeable membrane from an area of high solute concentration toward an area of low solute concentration is called
    A. diffusion
    B. facilitated diffusion
    C. active transport
    D. osmosis

16. Infusing a hypertonic solution into a blood vessel will cause all of the following to happen **EXCEPT**
    A. an osmotic gradient toward the vein
    B. a fluid shift into the blood vessel
    C. an increase in blood pressure
    D. a decrease in intravascular blood volume

17. A solution with the same osmolarity as blood plasma is said to be
    A. hypotonic
    B. hypertonic
    C. isotonic
    D. none of the above

18. In a fresh water drowning, what happens as water enters the pulmonary capillaries?
    A. It remains in the capillaries
    B. It quickly diffuses into the cells
    C. It draws additional fluid into the blood vessel
    D. None of the above

19. Sodium is transported out of the cell against the gradient in a process called
    A. facilitated diffusion
    B. facilitated transport
    C. passive diffusion
    D. active transport

20. The insulin/glucose relationship is an example of
    A. facilitated diffusion
    B. facilitated transport
    C. passive diffusion
    D. active transport

21. The majority of blood volume consists of

    A. red blood cells
    B. plasma
    C. platelets
    D. white blood cells

22. The percentage of red blood cells in the blood is called
    A. homeostasis
    B. hematocrit
    C. hemoglobin
    D. hematoma

23. Red blood cells make up what percentage of total blood volume in the healthy adult?
    A. 20
    B. 45
    C. 55
    D. 60

24. The universal recipient is blood type
    A. A
    B. B
    C. AB
    D. O

25. The universal donor is blood type
    A. A
    B. B
    C. AB
    D. O

26. A patient with blood infusing suddenly develops fever, chills, nausea, hives, tachycardia, and hypotension. You suspect a transfusion reaction. Which of the following should you do?
    A. Stop the IV
    B. Infuse normal saline
    C. Monitor the patient closely
    D. All of the above

27. Hespan, Dextran, and Albumin are examples of
    A. colloids
    B. crystalloids
    C. isotonic solutions
    D. hypotonic solutions

28. After infusing a colloid solution, you should expect
    A. a decrease in blood pressure
    B. a fluid shift into the bloodstream
    C. rapid diffusion of its solute particles into the tissues
    D. an osmotic gradient toward the intracellular compartment

29. How much Lactated Ringer's solution remains in the intravascular compartment after one hour?

    A. 100%
    B. 66%
    C. 50%
    D. 33%

30. The normal pH for the human body is
    A. 7.0-8.0
    B. 7.35-7.45
    C. 7.3
    D. 7.5

31. The fastest mechanism for correcting the body's acid-base abnormalities is the
    A. respiratory system
    B. renal system
    C. buffer system
    D. none of the above

32. A patient with a pH of 7.2 and a $PaCO_2$ of 52 torr is in a state of
    A. respiratory acidosis
    B. respiratory alkalosis
    C. metabolic acidosis
    D. metabolic alkalosis

33. A probable cause of this patient's condition is
    A. near drowning
    B. amphetamine drug overdose
    C. antacid ingestion
    D. excessive vomiting

34. The reasons behind the pH and $PaCO_2$ abnormalities include
    A. an increase in carbon dioxide elimination
    B. an increase in bicarbonate concentration
    C. a decrease in carbon dioxideretention
    D. none of the above

35. Immediate management of a patient in respiratory acidosis includes
    A. coaching the patient to breathe slower
    B. administration of sodium bicarbonate
    C. positive pressure ventilation
    D. none of the above

36. Which of the following is true regarding a patient in alkalosis?
    A. The pH is abnormally low
    B. The hydrogen ion concentration is abnormally high
    C. There are no bicarbonate ions present
    D. None of the above

37. Management of the patient in respiratory alkalosis includes
    A. hyperventilation
    B. coaching and reassurance
    C. breathing into a paper bag
    D. administration of sodium bicarbonate

38. The chief buffer of the acid-base system is
   A. phosphorus
   B. carbonic acid
   C. bicarbonate
   D. carbonic anhydrase

39. Which of the following factors **DOES NOT AFFECT** the heart's stroke volume?
   A. Heart rate
   B. Preload
   C. Afterload
   D. Contractile force

40. Preload could be increased by all of the following **EXCEPT**
   A. increasing venous return
   B. increasing contractile force
   C. decreasing afterload
   D. promoting venodilation

41. The amount of blood pumped from the heart in one contraction is called
   A. preload
   B. afterload
   C. stroke volume
   D. tidal volume

42. Which of the following statements best illustrates the Frank-Starling mechanism?
   A. The greater the afterload, the greater the stroke volume
   B. The less stroke volume, the less the afterload
   C. The greater the preload, the greater the stroke volume
   D. The less preload, the greater the afterload

43. In order to decrease the workload on the heart in a patient with CHF you should
   A. place the victim in Trendelenberg
   B. administer a drug that dilates the veins
   C. administer a fluid challenge
   D. hyperventilate the patient

44. The amount of blood pumped by the heart in one minute is called
   A. minute volume
   B. stroke volume
   C. cardiac output
   D. contractile volume

45. The amount of resistance against which the heart must pump in order to eject blood is called
   A. stroke volume
   B. end-diastolic volume
   C. afterload
   D. pulse pressure

46. Baroreceptors constantly monitor for changes in

    A. oxygen levels
    B. carbon dioxide levels
    C. heart rate
    D. blood pressure

47. Stimulation of the baroreceptors causes all of the following EXCEPT
    A. peripheral vasodilation
    B. increased cardiac output
    C. increased heart rate
    D. bronchodilation

48. Peripheral vascular resistance is dependent upon
    A. vessel diameter
    B. fluid viscosity
    C. vessel length
    D. all of the above

49. The greatest change in peripheral resistance occurs in the
    A. aorta
    B. arteries
    C. arterioles
    D. capillaries

50. Which of the following is a component of the "Fick Principle?"
    A. Adequate FiO_2
    B. Adequate hematocrit
    C. Adequate diffusion of gases
    D. All of the following

51. Anaerobic metabolism results in which of the following?
    A. Inefficient energy
    B. Increased pyruvic acid formation
    C. Glycolysis
    D. All of the above

52. Tachycardia, cool, clammy, and pale skin, and a stable blood pressure describes a patient in
    A. compensated shock
    B. decompensated shock
    C. irreversible shock
    D. none of the above

53. Which of the following happens in decompensated shock?
    A. Pre-capillary sphinctors open
    B. Rouleaux formation
    C. Blood pressure falls
    D. All of the above

54. In which of the following situations in the PASG CONTRAINDICATED?
    A. Suspected intra-abdominal hemorrhage
    B. Lower extremity hemorrhage
    C. Acute pulmonary edema secondary to cardiogenic shock
    D. Pelvic fracture

55. In a microdrip solution set, _____ drops equals 1 ml.
   A. 10
   B. 15
   C. 30
   D. 60

56. Through which of the following catheters can you deliver the most rapid fluid challenge?
   A. 12 gauge, 4 inch
   B. 12 gauge, 1 inch
   C. 24 gauge, 4 inch
   D. 24 gauge, 1 inch

57. Chills, fever, nausea, and vomiting following IV insertion indicates a/an
   A. inadvertent arterial puncture
   B. pyrogenic reaction
   C. thrombophlebitis
   D. air embolism

58. In this case you should immediately
   A. place the patient head down on his left side
   B. place warm packs on the IV site
   C. stop the IV
   D. clear the IV line of any air

59. The maximum amount of IV fluids that you should administer in the field is
   A. 1 liter
   B. 2-3 liters
   C. 5 liters
   D. none of the above

ANSWERS   **1. ANS—B**   *PEC—290*

Water is the most abundance substance in the human body. In fact, it counts for approximately 60% of the total body weight.

2. ANS—C   *PEC—291*

Approximately 75% of all body water is found within the intracellular compartment. This compartment is found inside the body's cells.

Body Fluid Compartments		
Compartment	Percentage of Total Body Water	Volume in 70 kg Adult
Intracellular Fluid	75%	31.50 L
Extracellular Fluid	25%	10.50 L
Interstitial Fluid	17.5%	7.35 L
Intravascular Fluid	7.5%	3.15 L

3. ANS—C   *PEC—292*

When your fluid levels drop, the pituitary gland at the base of the brain secrets the hormone ADH, or antidiuretic hormone. ADH causes the kidneys to reabsorb more water back into the bloodstream and excrete less urine.

4. ANS—B   *PEC—293*

Clinically, the dehydrated patient exhibits dry mucous membranes and poor skin turgor. As the dehydration becomes more severe, the pulse will quicken, and the blood pressure will drop. In infants, the anterior fontenal may be sunken.

5. ANS—D   *PEC—293*

Treatment for dehydration is fluid replacement. Since you cannot determine electrolyte deficits in the field, you should use isotonic solutions such as normal saline or Lactated Ringer's. For mild to moderate dehydration, run the infusion at 100-200 ml per hour.

6. ANS—C   *PEC—293*

The medication that stimulates the kidneys to excrete water is called a diuretic. An example of a diuretic is lasix or furosemide.

7. ANS—A   *PEC—293*

Electrolytes are substances that dissociate into charged particles when placed into water. Ions with a positive charge are called cations.

8. ANS—B   *PEC—293*

Sodium is the most prevalent cation in the extracellular fluid. It plays a major role in regulating the distribution of water.

9. ANS—C   *PEC—293*

Potassium is the most prevalent cation in the intracellular fluid. It plays an important role in the transmission of electrical impulses.

10. ANS—D   *PEC—293*

Calcium has many physiological functions. It plays a major role in muscular contraction as well as nerve impulse transmission.

11. ANS—A   *PEC—294*

Bicarbonate is the principal buffer of the body. It neutralizes the highly acidic hydrogen ion and other organic acids.

12. ANS—B   *PEC—294*

Electrolytes are usually measured in milliequivalents per liter—mEq/L.

13. ANS—D   *PEC—295*

Osmosis is the movement of water across a semipermeable membrane from an area of lesser solute concentration to an area of greater solute concentration. This movement occurs until the solute concentrations on both sides are equal.

Figure 12-1

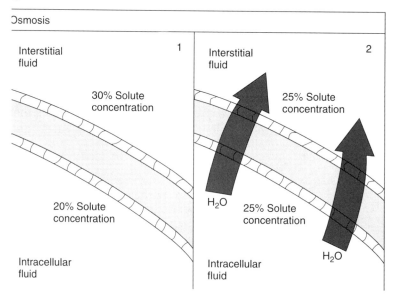

Source: PEC, Figure 12-4.

14. ANS—A   *PEC—295*

Infusing a hypotonic solution into the bloodstream causes water to move from
the bloodstream into the cells. This occurs because water tends to move from
areas of low solute concentration, which in this case will be the blood stream,
toward areas of higher solute concentration, which in this case will be the interstitial spaces and cells.

15. ANS—A   *PEC—294*

Diffusion is the movement of solutes from an area of greater concentration to
an area of lesser concentration. This movement occurs until the solute concentrations on both sides are equal.

Figure 12-2

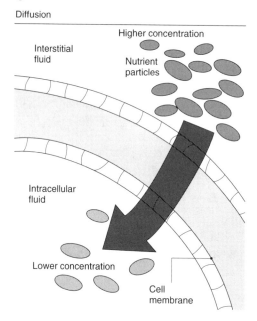

Source: PEC, Figure 12-3.

16. ANS—D   *PEC—295*

Infusing a hypertonic solution into a blood vessel will cause an osmotic gradient which shifts water into the blood vessel. This will cause an increase in blood pressure.

17. ANS—C   *PEC—294*

A solution with the same osmolarity as blood plasma is isotonic. Isotonic is a state in which solutions on opposite sides of a semipermeable membrane are in equal concentration.

18. ANS—B   *PEC—294*

In a fresh water drowning, water enters the pulmonary capillaries and quickly diffuses into the cells. This occurs because fresh water is hypotonic.

19. ANS—D   *PEC—296*

Sodium is transported out of the cell by a process called active transport. Active transport is a biochemical process in which substances use energy to move across the cell membrane against the normal gradiant. Active transport is faster than diffusion, but it requires the expenditure of energy.

20. ANS—A   *PEC—296*

The insulin-glucose relationship is an example of facilitated diffusion. Facili- ated diffusion is a biochemical process in which a substance is selectively trans- ported across a membrane using helper proteins and requires energy.

21. ANS—B   *PEC—297*

Plasma makes up approximately 55% of the total blood volume. It consists of 92% water, 6-7% proteins, and a small portion consisting of electrolytes, lipids, enzymes, clotting factors, glucose, and other dissolved substances.

22. ANS—B   *PEC—297*

The percentage of blood occupied by red blood cells is referred to as the hema- tocrit. Normal hematocrit in the healthy person is approximately 45%.

23. ANS—B   *PEC—297*

Red blood cells account for approximately 45% of the total blood volume. This percentage is known as the patient's hematocrit.

24. ANS—C   *PEC—298*

Persons with type AB blood are referred to as universal recipients. These peo- ple do not have antibodies to either A or B since they carry both antigens. In an emergency, they can receive blood of any type.

Blood Typing—ABO System		
Blood Type	**Antigen Present on RBC**	**Antibody Present in Serum**
0	None	Anti-A, Anti-B
AB	A and B	None
B	B	Anti-A
A	A	Anti-B

25. ANS—D *PEC—298*

Type O blood does not contain either the A or B antigen. In an emergency, it can be administered to a patient of any blood type. Because of this, type O is referred to as the universal donor.

Compatibility Among ABO Blood Groups				
	Reaction with Serum of Recipient			
Cells of Donor	AB	B	A	O
AB	−	+	+	+
B	−	−	+	+
A	−	+	−	+
O	−	−	−	−
− = Nonagglutination				
+ = Agglutination				

26. ANS—D *PEC—299*

Signs and symptoms of a transfusion reaction include fever, chills, hives, hypotension, palpitations, tachycardia, flushing of the skin, headaches, loss of consciousness, nausea and vomiting, and shortness of breath. If you suspect a transfusion reaction, stop the IV, infuse normal saline, and monitor the patient closely.

27. ANS—A *PEC—301*

Hespan, Dextran, and Albumin are examples of colloids. Colloids are solutions that contain proteins or other high molecular weight molecules that tend to remain in the intravascular space for an extended period of time.

28. ANS—B *PEC—301*

Colloids create a colloid osmotic pressure and tend to attract water into the intravascular space. Colloids draw water from the interstitial spaces and the intracellular compartment in order to increase the intravascular blood volume.

29. AND—D *PEC—302*

Due to the movement of the electrolytes and water, two-thirds of crystalloid solutions such as Lactated Ringer's and normal saline is lost to the interstitial space within one hour.

30. ANS—B *PEC—302*

The normal pH for the human body is 7.35—7.45.

31. ANS—C *PEC—303*

There are three major mechanisms to remove acids from the body. The fastest mechanism is often referred to as the buffer system, or the bicarbonate buffer system. This system works in seconds.

32. ANS—A PEC—305

A patient with a pH of 7.2 and a $PaCO_2$ of 52 torr is in a state of respiratory acidosis.

33. ANS—A PEC—305

A probable cause for this patient's condition could be a near-drowning. Respiratory acidosis is caused by the retention of carbon dioxide. This can result from impaired ventilation due to problems occuring in either the lungs or in the respiratory center of the brain.

34. ANS—D *PEC—305*

The reasons behind this patient's pH and PCO2 levels include a decrease in carbon dioxide elimination and an increase in carbon dioxide retention.

35. ANS—C *PEC—305*

Immediate management of the patient in respiratory acidosis is aimed at improving ventilation and oxygenation. Vigorously ventilate this patient with positive pressure and 100% oxygen.

36. ANS—D *PEC—305*

Alkalosis is a state in which the patient's hyrodgen ion concentration is abnormally low and the pH is high.

37. ANS—B *PEC—305*

Management of a patient in respiratory alkalosis is aimed at helping the patient retain carbon dioxide. Respiratory alkalosis results from the excessive elimination of carbon dioxide. This can occur with anxiety or following climbing to a high altitude. It can also occur as a compensatory mechanism in shock and a variety of other serious hypoxic conditions. For this reason, withholding oxygen from this patient could prove to be a fatal mistake. Simply place your patient on a rebreather mask with 10-15 lpm. oxygen flow and coach him to breathe slowly.

38. ANS—C *PEC—303*

The chief buffer of the acid base system is bicarbonate.

39. ANS—A *PEC—307*

The amount of blood ejected by the heart at one contraction is referred to as the stroke volume. Stroke volume is determined by preload, afterload, and contractile force.

40. ANS—D *PEC—308*

Preload could be increased by increasing venous return, by increasing contractile force of the heart, and by decreasing the afterload.

41. ANS—C *PEC—307*

The amount of blood pumped from the heart in one contraction is called stroke volume.

42. ANS—C *PEC—308*

The greater the volume of preload the more the ventricles are stretched. The greater the stretch, up to a certain point, the greater the subsequent cardiac contraction. This is referred to as the Frank-Starling mechanism.

43. ANS—B PEC—307

For a patient in severe congestive heart failure you want to decrease the workload on the heart by decreasing preload. You could accomplish this by administering drugs such as nitroglycerin, furosemide, and morphine which dilate the veins. Dilating the veins causes pooling of blood on the venous side and decreases preload.

44. ANS—C   *PEC—308*

The amount of blood pumped from the heart in one minute is called cardiac output. Cardiac output is calculated by stroke volume times heart rate.

45. ANS—C   *PEC—308*

The amount of resistance against which the heart must pump is called afterload. The heart must overcome this resistance in order to eject blood. Afterload is determined by the degree of peripheral vascular resistance. Peripheral resistance is determined by the degree of vasoconstriction present on the arterial side.

46. ANS—D   *PEC—308*

Baroreceptors are located in the carotid bodies and the arch of the aorta. These baroreceptors closely monitor pressure.

47. ANS—A   *PEC—308*

Baroreceptors are stretch receptors that stretch with increased pressure. When they detect reduced flow and pressure they send messages to the brain to stimulate the sympathetic nervous system. This results in increased heart rate and cardiac output to increase circulation and bronchodilation

48. ANS—D   *PEC—309*

Blood flow through a blood vessel is determined by peripheral resistence and pressure within the system. Peripheral resistance is defined as resistance to blood flow and is dependent upon three factors, the length of the vessel, the diameter of the vessel, and blood viscosity.

49. ANS—C   *PEC—309*

There is very little resistance to blood flow through the aorta and arteries. A significant change in peripheral resistance occurs at the arteriole level. This is because the inside diameter of the arteriole is much smaller as compared to the aorta and arteries. Additionally, the arteriole has pronounced ability to change its diameter as much as five-fold in response to local tissue needs and autonomic nervous system signals.

50. ANS—D   *PEC—310*

The movement and utilization of oxygen in the body depends upon the following conditions: adequate concentration of inspired oxygen; appropriate movement of oxygen across the alveolar-capillary membrane into the bloodstream; adequate number of red blood cells to carry the oxygen; proper tissue perfusion, and efficient off-loading of oxygen at the tissue level. These conditions are collectively known as the Fick Principle.

51. ANS—D   *PEC—311*

During periods of inadquate tissue perfusion, cell metabolism switches from aerobic to an anaerobic mode. Results of this process are inefficient energy, an increase in pyruvic acid formation, and glycoloysis.

52. ANS—A   *PEC—313*

Following the onset of inadequate tissue perfusion, various compensatory mechanisms of the body are stimulated. The heart rate and strength of cardiac contractions increase. There will be an increase in systemic vascular resistance to assist in maintaining the blood pressure. These compensatory changes will continue until the body is unable to maintain blood pressure and tissue perfusion. Your patient in compensatory shock will exhibit tachycardia, cool, clammy, and pale skin with a stable blood pressure.

53. ANS—D   *PEC—313*

In the later stages of shock the blood pressure begins to fall and blood supply to essential organs diminishes. As a result, the pre-capillary sphinctors open while the post-capillary sphinctors remain closed. This results in sludging of red blood cells and the formation of rouleaux.

54. ANS—C   *PEC—322*

Application of the pneumatic anti-shock garment is contraindicated in the presence of pulmonary edema occuring secondary to heart failure. This is because adding fluid volume to the central circulation and increasing afterload may further compromise an already failing heart.

55. ANS—D   *PEC—326*

In a microdrip solution set, 60 drops equals 1 ml.

56. ANS—B   *PEC—326*

In order to infuse the most fluid the most rapidly, use the largest diameter cannula with the shortest possible needle length.

57. ANS—B   *PEC—330*

A pyrogenic reaction occurs when pyrogens "foreign particles capable of producing fever" are present in the administration set or intravenous solution. It is characterized by the abrupt onset of fever, chills, backache, headache, nausea, and vomiting. Cardiovascular collapse may also result.

58. ANS—C   *PEC—330*

In a case of pyrogenic reaction terminate the IV immediately and establish another IV in the other arm using a new administration set and solution.

59. ANS—B   *PEC—331*

The maximum amount of intravenous fluids that should be administered to an adult in the field setting is about 2-3 liters. More than 2-3 liters of fluid therapy would reduce the hematocrit to the point of being ineffective.

CHAPTER 13

Emergency Pharmacology

QUESTIONS

1. Atropine and digitalis are examples of drugs derived from
   A. plants
   B. minerals
   C. animals
   D. synthetics

2. Insulin and pitocin are examples of drugs derived from
   A. plants
   B. minerals
   C. animals
   D. synthetics

3. Calcium chloride and sodium bicarbonate are examples of drugs derived from
   A. plants
   B. minerals
   C. animals
   D. synthetics

4. Lidocaine and procainamide are examples of drugs derived from
   A. plants
   B. minerals
   C. animals
   D. synthetics

5. The Federal Food, Drug, and Cosmetic Act of 1938 required that
  A. all ingredients be placed on the label
  B. all opium by-products be classified according to schedules
  C. all prescriptions be filled within 72 hours
  D. all of the above

6. The Harrison Narcotic Act of 1914 regulates the sale of
  A. cocaine
  B. morphine
  C. all drugs
  D. barbiturates and amphetamines

7. The Controlled Substances Act of 1970 established
  A. schedules for abusive drugs
  B. time limits for filling prescriptions
  C. no refills for classified drugs
  D. all of the above

8. Furosemide, diazepam, and meperidine are examples of
  A. chemical names
  B. trade names
  C. brand names
  D. generic names

9. Lasix, Valium, and Demerol are examples of
  A. trade names
  B. chemical names
  C. official names
  D. generic names

10. The PDR is a useful tool for identifying drugs by
  A. name
  B. size
  C. color
  D. all of the above

11. D_5W and Lactated Ringer's are examples of
  A. tinctures
  B. suspensions
  C. solutions
  D. emulsions

12. Iodine and merthiolate are examples of
  A. tinctures
  B. suspensions
  C. emulsions
  D. elixirs

13. Amoxicillin and calamine lotion are examples of
  A. emulsions
  B. spirits
  C. suspensions
  D. solutions

14. Ammonia capsules are examples of
  A. emulsions
  B. spirits
  C. suspensions
  D. tinctures

15. Oil and water form a/an
  A. solution
  B. emulsion
  C. elixir
  D. spirit

16. The difference between a syrup and an elixir is that
  A. elixirs contain alcohol and flavoring
  B. syrups contain alcohol and flavoring
  C. elixirs contain drugs suspended in sugar and water
  D. none of the above

17. Which of the following is NOT an example of a drug administered parenterally?
  A. Intramuscular (IM)
  B. Intravenously (IV)
  C. Subcutaneously (SC)
  D. Orally (PO)

18. The action of naloxone on morphine is an example of
  A. synergism
  B. antagonism
  C. cumulative action
  D. potentiation

19. Repeating boluses of lidocaine until the desired effect is reached is an example of
  A. synergism
  B. potentiation
  C. cumulative action
  D. agonism

20. The enhancing effect of taking barbiturates with alcohol is an example of
  A. antagonism
  B. potentiation
  C. synergism
  D. cumulative action

21. Using albuterol and aminophylline to dilate the airways is an example of
  A. potentiation
  B. cumulative action
  C. antagonism
  D. synergism

22. A patient who once took 5 mg of diazepam each day now requires 10 mg. This is an example of
  A. potentiation
  B. tolerance

    C. becoming refractory
    D. untoward effect

23. An individual reaction to a drug that is unusually different from that normally seen is called a/an
    A. hypersensitivity
    B. idiosyncrasy
    C. adverse reaction
    D. untoward effect

24. Isoproterenol is not given in cardiac arrest because it is
    A. indicated
    B. potentiated
    C. synergistic
    D. contraindicated

25. Which of the following will affect a drug's rate of absorption?
    A. Circulation
    B. Patient size and age
    C. General medical condition
    D. All of the above

26. Which of the following has the quickest absorption?
    A. Intramuscular (IM)
    B. Subcutaneously (SC)
    C. Intravenously (IV)
    D. Orally (PO)

27. Which of the following is true regarding drug distribution?
    A. Binding to proteins normally produces a delayed onset
    B. Rapid onset usually means short duration
    C. Organs with the best circulation, get the most drug concentration
    D. All of the above

28. If drug X is a weak penetrator of the blood brain barrier,
    A. it is probably not protein bound
    B. it is probably ionized
    C. it is not ionized
    D. none of the above

29. The process of changing a drug to another form, either active or inactive, is known as
    A. distribution
    B. metabolism
    C. biotransformation
    D. pharmacokinetics

30. Drugs that bind to a receptor and produce a response are known as
    A. antagonists
    B. agonists
    C. biotransformers
    D. lytics

31. Drugs that bind to a receptor and block a response are known as
   A. antagonists
   B. agonists
   C. inhibitors
   D. mimetics

32. Drugs with a low therapeutic index
   A. are difficult to titrate
   B. have a narrow therapeutic range
   C. are easy to overdose
   D. all of the above

33. The sympathetic nervous system is responsible for
   A. vegetative functions
   B. custodial functions
   C. "feeding and breeding"
   D. the stress response

34. When stimulated, the sympathetic nervous system causes all of the following physiological responses EXCEPT
   A. pupil dilation
   B. peripheral vasodilation
   C. increased cardiac contractions
   D. increased heart rate

35. The sympathetic receptors are activated by the neurotransmitter
   A. acetylcholine
   B. insulin
   C. norepinephrine
   D. dopamine

36. Which of the following adrenergic receptors causes bronchodilation and peripheral vasodilation when stimulated?
   A. Beta 1
   B. Beta 2
   C. Alpha 1
   D. Dopaminergic

37. Drugs that stimulate the sympathetic nervous system are called
   A. sympathomimetics
   B. sympatholytics
   C. beta blockers
   D. alpha antagonists

38. Stimulating the dopaminergic receptors causes
   A. increased heart rate
   B. peripheral vasoconstriction
   C. renal, coronary, and cerebral artery vasodilation
   D. bronchodilation, vasodilation, and pupil constriction

39. Which receptors cause peripheral vasoconstriction?
   A. Beta 1
   B. Beta 2

    C. Alpha 1

    D. Dopaminergic

40. Which receptors would stimulate the heart to beat faster and stronger?

    A. Beta 1

    B. Beta 2

    C. Alpha 1

    D. Dopaminergic

41. The parasympathetic nervous system is responsible for

    A. "feeding and breeding"

    B. resting heart rate

    C. digestion

    D. all of the above

42. The parasympathetic nervous system exerts its control via

    A. several cranial nerves

    B. vagus nerve

    C. some sacral nerves

    D. all of the above

43. The parasympathetic nervous system uses the neurotransmitter

    A. norepinephrine

    B. epinephrine

    C. acetylcholine

    D. cholinesterase

44. When stimulated, the parasympathetic receptors cause

    A. decreased salivation

    B. pupil dilation

    C. increased heart rate

    D. none of the above

45. An example of a parasympatholytic is

    A. epinephrine

    B. propranolol

    C. atropine

    D. acetylcholine

46. Intradermal drugs are most commonly used for

    A. shock

    B. diagnostic testing

    C. prophylaxis

    D. respiratory emergencies

47. Nitroglycerine patches are examples of _____ medications.

    A. intradermal

    B. transtracheal

    C. subcutaneous

    D. transdermal

48. A subcutaneous injection is administered at a _____ angle to the skin.

    A. 45°

    B. 90°

    C. 180°

    D. 5°

49. An intramuscular injection is administered at a _____ angle to the skin.

    A. 45°

    B. 90°

    C. 180°

    D. 5°

50. It is important to aspirate for blood return when administering medications via the IM route to ensure

    A. the airway is patent

    B. the needle is in a vein

    C. the needle is in the artery

    D. the needle is not in a blood vessel

51. Which of the following inhaled medications has B-2 receptor preference and is effective in relieving subglottic edema?

    A. albuterol

    B. oxygen

    C. vaponefrin

    D. atrovent

52. Which of the following is a calcium channel blocker?

    A. Procardia

    B. Adenocard

    C. Furosemide

    D. Levophed

53. Which of the following inhaled medications is a parasympathetic agent that also dries respiratory secretions?

    A. albuterol

    B. oxygen

    C. vaponefrin

    D. atrovent

54. A 40-year-old male presents lethargic with slurred speech. Evaluation reveals bilateral weakness. His son relates the patient is a diabetic and a fingerstick reveals a blood glucose level of 20. Several intravenous attempts are unsuccessful due to the patient's uncooperative behavior; what drug would you administer next?

    A. glucose gel sublingually

    B. D50 intramuscularly

    C. Glucagon 0.3 mg intramuscularly

    D. Glucagon 1.0 mg intramuscularly

    E. transport guarding the patient's airway and do nothing else

55. True or False:

Adenosine is administered slow IV push.

56. True or False:

Atropine is indicated for bradycardia associated with Type II (Mobitz) and Type III AV block.

57. Which is the preferred vasopressor for treating cardiogenic shock?
   A. Dopamine
   B. Dobutamine
   C. Norepinephrine
   D. Epinephrine

58. Dopamine at doses greater than 20 mcg/kg/min affects which receptors predominately?
   A. beta-1
   B. alpha
   C. dopaminergic
   D. beta-2

59. The following medications slow AV conduction. Which one is an endogenous nucleoside?
   A. Isoptin
   B. Adenocard
   C. Digoxin
   D. Procainamide

60. Which class of pharmaceuticals is contraindicated in asthma?
   A. beta blockers
   B. calcium channel blockers
   C. xanthines
   D. diuretics

61. Which inhaled medication can cause altered mental status?
   A. Nitronox
   B. Vaponefrin
   C. Atrovent
   D. Ventolin

62. You are called to evaluate a 30-month-old child with a barking cough that has worsened all day. The patient appears in moderate to severe distress. The best medication to remediate this problem is
   A. oxygen
   B. albuterol nebulizer
   C. ipatroprium nebulizer
   D. vaponefrin nebulizer

63. A 40-year-old man is found by the paramedics to be aphasic with his head turned to the left and his eyes stuck in extreme upward and lateral gaze. His wife notes he has used a suppository recently to control his nausea after dental surgery. Which medication would you consider administering?
   A. Narcan
   B. Benadryl
   C. Phenergan
   D. Thiamine

64. All of the following are sympathomimetics except
   A. Adrenaline
   B. Levophed

    C. Normodyne
    D. Intropin

65. Which of the following drugs is an antiarrhythmic?
    A. Haldol
    B. Labetolol
    C. SoluMedrol
    D. Bretylol

66. All of the following are deactivated by higher pH except
    A. Norepinephrine
    B. Dopamine
    C. Epinephrine
    D. Sodium Bicarbonate

67. Which of the following statements regarding Lidocaine is true?
    A. it accelerates depolarization and automaticity in the ventricles
    B. it effects the aria more than the ventricles
    C. it increases the fibrillation threshold
    D. it slows atrioventricular conduction
    E. it depresses myocardial contractility

68. All of the following are considered malignant premature ventricular contractions except
    A. multifocal PVC's
    B. couplets
    C. R on T phenomena
    D. more than ten per minute

69. True or False

Lidocaine is contraindicated in second degree Type II and third degree antrioventricular block.

70. True or False

When bradycardia and PVC's occur together, the PVC's should be treated first.

71. Caution must be used when using Levophed concomitantly with what class of drugs as it can precipitate a rise in blood pressue?
    A. beta blockers
    B. calcium channel blockers
    C. alpha blockers
    D. anticholinergics

72. The dose of Lidocaine is
    A. 1.0–1.5 gm/kg initially
    B. 0.1–1.5 mg/kg initially
    C. 1.0–1.5 mg/kg initially
    D. repeated every ten minutes at half the initial dose

73. The following drugs can be administered endotracheally except
    A. xylocaine
    B. naloxone

    C. adrenalin

    D. adenocard

74. Which of the following is derived from the belladonna plant?

    A. morphine sulfate

    B. digoxin

    C. atropine sulfate

    D. adenosine

75. All of the following cause potential hypotension except

    A. labetolol

    B. dobutamine

    C. procainamide

    D. bretylium

76. Which of the following calcium channel blockers acts primarily in the peripheral vasculature and does not slow AV conduction?

    A. Procardia

    B. Calan

    C. Cardizem

    D. Verapamil

77. A 38-year-old primipara female who is in the 36th week of gestation is complaining of marked weakness and swelling of her extremities. Secondary examination reveals she has an elevated blood pressure. On the way to the hospital the patient begins to seize. What is your drug of choice?

    A. valium

    B. magnesium sulfate

    C. morphine sulfate

    D. oxytocin

Match the following mediation with its action:

78. dobutamine	**A.**	has alpha and beta effects but more so stimulates beta receptors
79. dopamine	**B.**	a positive inotrope, a dose-related chronotrope
80. norepinephrine	**C.**	has alpha and beta effects but more so stimulates alpha receptors
81. epinephrine	**D.**	a positive inotrope, little chronotropy.

82. A 49-year-old male presents in respiratory arrest as you find him slumped in his car. The patient is not wearing a shirt and you notice multiple blisters and scars on his forearms. The patient's airway is clear and BLS crews are easily ventilating the patient with a bag-valve-mask and oropharyngeal airway. Your next step is to use

    A. dextrose

    B. thiamine

   C. narcan

   D. valium

83. The initial dose of the medication chosen above is

   A. 1.0 gram

   B. 100 milligrams

   C. 10 milligrams

   D. 2.0 milligrams

84. The following routes may be used to administer this drug except

   A. PO

   B. IV

   C. ETT

   D. SQ

85. Which of the following medications is used for ventricular arrhythmia and also has obstetrical indications

   A. bretylium tosylate

   B. morphine sulfate

   C. oxytocin

   D. magnesium sulfate

86. Which of the following medications is used both to induce labor and also to stop postpartum hemorrhage

   A. magnesium sulfate

   B. pitocin

   C. terbutaline

   D. brethine

87. All of the following are side effects of magnesium sulfate except

   A. arrhythmia

   B. respiratory depression

   C. hypotension

   D. increased deep tendon reflexes

88. Syrup of Ipecac is classified as a/an

   A. emetic

   B. adsorbent

   C. antihistamine

   D. antiarrythmic

89. The pediatric dose of activated charcoal is

   A. 1 mg/kg

   B. 10 mg/kg

   C. 100 mg/kg

   D. 1000 mg/kg

90. All of the following are indications for using sodium bicarbonate except

   A. late in the management of cardiac arrest

   B. hypokalemia

   C. phenobarbitol overdose

   D. tricyclic antidepressant overdose

91. The initial dose of sodium bicarbonate is
A. 1.0 gram/kg
B. 0.1 gm/kg
C. 0.01 gm/kg
D. 0.001 gm/kg

92. Of the following narcotic medications, which has a dosing regimen that is essentially determined by the patient's self administration
A. nitronox
B. morphine
C. nubain
D. demerol

93. The route of choice to administer Lasix in an emergency is
A. orally
B. sublingually
C. endotracheally
D. intravenously

94. A 72-year-old female presents with a history of increasing shortness of breath, dyspnea on exertion. She denies having any chest pain or pressure. She had an MI five years ago and her only medication is Lopressor. Your examination reveals a third heart sound, increased jugular venous distention and peripheral edema. All of the following are indicated in the management of this patient except
A. morphine
B. furosemide
C. nitroglycerin
D. nifedipine

95. A 60-year-old man was driving on the expressway when he lost control of his car and drove into the median. He struck the steering wheel and complains of moderate chest pain. He appears anxious and describes the pain as similar to his heart attack of last year. History reveals he has stopped smoking since his MI and he takes an aspirin a day. Examination reveals a contusion over his sternum and tenderness on the left side of his chest. All of the following may be administered as needed except
A. morphine
B. nitroglycerin
C. nitrous oxide
D. oxygen

96. An 18-year-old female presents complaining of chest pain for the last four hours. It is associated with diaphoresis, nausea, and shortness of breath. She appears anxious. She is a smoker and finally revealed the symptoms began while she was smoking crack cocaine. Her vitals are HR 110, BP 120/65, RR 22. What medication would be best suited to administer to this patient?
A. nitroglycerin
B. nifedipine
C. oxygen
D. morphine

97. All of the following mechanisms pertaining to calcium chloride are true except
  A. increases myocardial contractile force
  B. increased ventricular automaticity
  C. used as an antidote for morphine sulfate toxicity
  D. can minimize side effects of calcium channel blocker usage

98. Choose the incorrect statement as it relates to calcium chloride
  A. it will precipitate with sodium bicarbonate
  B. it is used in the management of hyperkalemia and hypocalcemia problems
  C. it can lower digoxin levels therefore patients on digoxin will require higher doses
  D. it can cause arrhythmias, syncope, nausea, and cardiac arrest

99. All of the following statements regarding aminophylline are true except
  A. besides asthma, it is also useful in treating pesticide poisioning and emphysema
  B. concomitant use with beta blockers or erythromycin can cause theophylline toxicity
  C. it works by relaxing smooth muscles of the bronchioles without affecting adrenergic receptors
  D. it should not be used in patients with PVC's, tachycardia, or hypotension

100. True or False

Nitroglycerin should not be administered in all of the following scenarios:
  A. hypotensive patients
  B. patients who are allergic to nitrates
  C. patients with increased intracranial pressure
  D. patients who are in shock

Make the following conversions:

101. 3 kilograms   =   _____ grams

102. 2.5 grams   =   _____ milligrams

103. 8 milligrams   =   _____ micrograms

104. 3000 milliliters   =   _____ liters

105. 1/4 grain   =   _____ milligrams

106. 22 lb.   =   _____ kilograms

107. 800 micrograms   =   _____ milligrams

108. 3 liters   =   _____ milliliters

109. 500 milligrams   =   _____ grams

110. 5 grams   =   _____ micrograms

Calculate the following drug orders:

	Drug Order	Patient Weight	Administer
111.	1mg/kg	176 lbs.	_____ mg
112.	10mg/kg	220 lbs.	_____ mg
113.	20ml/kg	55 lbs.	_____ ml
114.	5mcg/kg/min	110 lbs.	_____ mcg/min
115.	0.1mg/kg	10 lbs.	_____ mg

Determine the following drug concentrations:

116.	100mg/10ml	_____/ml
117.	50mg/2ml	_____/ml
118.	250mg/20ml	_____/ml
119.	1 gram/10ml	_____/ml
120.	1mg/ml	_____/ml

Calculate the following drug administrations:

	Drug on Hand	Physician Order	Administer
121.	100mg/5ml	75mg	_____ ml
122.	1mg/ml	0.25mg	_____ ml
123.	50mg/2ml	25mg	_____ ml
124.	200mg/5ml	50mg	_____ ml
125.	1mg/10ml	0.5mg	_____ ml
126.	500mg/10ml	5mg/kg (198 lbs)	_____ ml
127.	100mg/10ml	1mg/kg (187 lbs)	_____ ml
128.	2mg/ml	10mg	_____ ml
129.	40mg/10ml	120mg	_____ ml
130.	400mg/20ml	80mg	_____ ml

Calculate the following drip rates using microdrip solution sets (60 drops/ml):

	Drug	Solution	MD Order	Drip Rate
131.	1 gram	250 ml	3 mg/min	_____ drops/min
132.	2 grams	500 ml	2 mg/min	_____ drops/min
133.	1 mg	250 ml	4 mcg/min	_____ drops/min
134.	400 mg	500 ml	5 mcg/kg/min (176 lbs.)	_____ drops/min
135.	1 gram	500 ml	2 mg/min	_____ drops/min

ANSWERS   **1. ANS—A**   *PEC—336*

Atropine and digitalis are examples of drugs derived from plants.

2. ANS—C   *PEC—336*

Insulin and pitocin are examples of drugs derived from animals.

3. ANS—B   *PEC—336*

Calcium chloride and sodium bicarbonate are examples of drugs derived from minerals.

4. ANS—D   *PEC—336*

Lidocaine and procainamide are examples of drugs derived from synthetics.

5. ANS—A   *PEC—337*

The Federal Food, Drug, and Cosmetic Act of 1938 requires the names of all ingredients of foods and medications to be placed on the product label. It also requires that the labels state whether the ingredients are habit forming and site the percentages of those drugs present.

6. ANS—B   *PEC—337*

The Harrison Narcotic Act of 1915 regulates the sale, importation, and manufacture of the opium plant and its derivatives.

7. ANS—D   *PEC—337*

In 1970, the government regulated addictive medications through the Controlled Substances Act. This act classifies addictive medications into five schedules, prohibited the refilling of prescriptions for schedule 2 drugs, and requires that the original prescription be filled within 72 hours.

8. ANS—D   *PEC—338*

Furosemide, diazepam, and meperidine are all examples of generic names. The generic name is the name usually given to a drug by its first manufacturer and is an abbreviated version of the chemical name.

9. ANS—A   *PEC—338*

Lasix, Valium, and Demerol are examples of trade names. The trade name is a name given to a drug by each manufacturer. A medication may appear under several trade names if it is made by a number of manufacturers.

10. ANS—D   *PEC—338*

The Physician's Desk Reference identifies drugs by name, size, and color. It is published yearly by the Medical Economics Company.

11. ANS—C   *PEC—339*

D5W and Lactated Ringer's are examples of solutions. Solutions are preparations in which the drugs are dissolved in a solvent, usually water.

12. ANS—A   *PEC—339*

Iodine and merthiolate are examples of tinctures. Tinctures are drug preparations in which the drug was extracted chemically with alcohol.

13. ANS—C   *PEC—339*

Amoxicillin and calamine lotion are examples of suspensions. Suspensions are liquid drug preparations that do not remain dissolved. After sitting for even a short time, these preparations will tend to separate. They must always be shaken well before use.

14. ANS—B *PEC—339*

Ammonia capsules are examples of spirits. Spirit solutions contain volatile chemicals dissolved in alcohol. These chemicals quickly vaporize when they hit the air.

15. ANS—B *PEC—339*

Oil and water form an emulsion. Emulsions are preparations in which an oily substance is mixed with a solvent that will not dissolve it. After mixing, globules of fat form and float in the solvent. These preparations are similar to what occurs in a mixture of oil and vinegar.

16. ANS—A *PEC—339*

Elixirs are preparations that contain the drug in an alcohol solution with an added flavoring to improve the taste. Syrups are drugs suspended in sugar and water to improve the taste.

17. ANS—D *PEC—339*

Liquid drugs administered into the body through intramuscular, subcutaneous, or intravenous routes are called parenteral drugs. These drugs are introduced into the body outside the digestive tract.

18. ANS—B *PEC—340*

The action of naloxone and morphine is an example of antagonism. Antagonism signifies the opposition between two or more medications. The two drugs compete for the limited number of receptor sites.

19. ANS—C *PEC—340*

Repeating boluses of lidocaine until the desired effect is reached is an example of cumulative action. This occurs when a drug is administered in several doses causing an increasing effect usually due to a build up of the drug in the blood.

20. ANS—B *PEC—340*

Enhancing the effect of taking barbiturates with alcohol is an example of potentiation. Potentiation is the enhancement of one drug's effects by another.

21. ANS—D *PEC—340*

Using albuterol and aminophylline to dilate the airways is an example of synergism. Synergism is the combined action of two drugs with different effects. The resulting effect is much stronger that the effects of either one separately.

22. ANS—B *PEC—340*

A patient who requires a higher dose of the same medication to reach the desired effect is an example of tolerance.

23. ANS—B *PEC—340*

An idiosyncrasy is an individual reaction to a drug that is unusually different from that normally seen.

24. ANS—D *PEC—340*

Contraindications are the medical or physiological conditions present in a patient that would make it harmful to administer an otherwise appropriate medication.

25. ANS—D   *PEC—341*

A drug's rate of absorption will be affected by the patient's circulatory status, size and age, and general medical condition.

26. ANS—C   *PEC—341*

The intravenous route has the quickest absorption rate because the drug is injected directly into the circulatory system through the veins.

27. ANS—D   *PEC—341*

Drugs that bind to proteins normally produce a delayed onset. Drugs with a rapid onset usually have a short duration and organs with the best circulation get the most drug concentration.

28. ANS—B   *PEC—342*

Drugs that are protein bound or drugs in an ionized form are weak penetrators of the blood-brain barrier.

29. ANS—C   *PEC—342*

The process of changing a drug to another form, either active or inactive, is called biotransformation. It results in chemical variations of the drug which are called metabolites.

30. ANS—B   *PEC—343*

Drugs that bind to a receptor and produce a response are known as agonists. An example is epinephrine which stimulates the alpha and beta receptors in the heart, blood vessels, and lower airways.

Figure 13-1

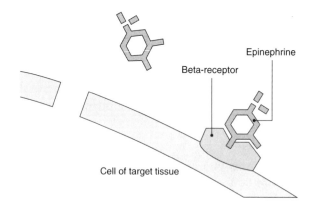

Source: PEC, Figure 13-5.

31. ANS—A   *PEC—343*

Drugs that bind to a receptor and block a response are known as antagonists. An example is naloxone which blocks the narcotic receptor sites.

Figure 13-2

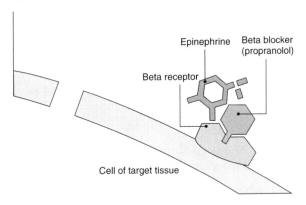

Source: PEC, Figure 13-6.

32. ANS—D   *PEC—344*

Drugs with a low therapeutic index are difficult to titrate because they have a narrow therapeutic range. It is very easy to overdose patients on these types of drugs.

Figure 13-3

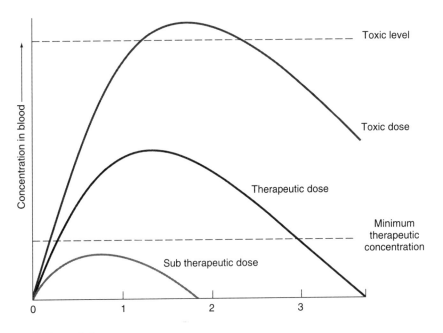

Source: PEC, Figure 13-7.

33. ANS—D   *PEC—347*

The sympathetic nervous system allows the body to function under stress. It is also referred to as the fight/flight aspect of the nervous system when stimulated.

34. ANS—B   *PEC—347*

When stimulated, the sympathetic nervous system causes pupillary dilation, an increase in heart rate, an increase in the force of cardiac contractions, peripheral vasoconstriction, and increased metabolic rate.

35. ANS—C   *PEC—348*

The sympathetic receptors are activated by the neurotransmitter norepinephrine.

36. ANS—B   *PEC—349*

When the beta 2 receptors are stimulated, bronchodilation and peripheral vasodilation occur.

37. ANS—A   *PEC—349*

Drugs that stimulate the sympathetic nervous system are called sympathomimetics. Examples include epinephrine, isoproterenol, dopamine, and norepinephrine.

38. ANS—C   *PEC—349*

Stimulating the dopaminergic receptors causes renal, coronary, and cerebral artery vasodilation.

39. ANS—C   *PEC—349*

When the alpha receptors are stimulated, peripheral vasoconstriction occurs.

40. ANS—A   *PEC—349*

When the beta 1 receptors are stimulated, the heart beats faster and stronger.

41. ANS—D   *PEC—350*

The parasympathetic nervous system primarily controls vegetative functions such as digestion of food and resting heart rate. It is often referred to as the "feed or breed" aspect of the autonomic nervous system.

42. ANS—D   *PEC—350*

The parasympathetic nervous system exerts it control via several cranial nerves, primarily the vagus nerve, and some sacral nerves.

43. ANS—C   *PEC—351*

The parasympathetic nervous system uses the neurotransmitter acetylcholine.

44. ANS—D   *PEC—351*

When stimulated, the parasympathetic nervous system decreases the heart rate, promotes increased salivation, and causes pupillary constriction.

45. ANS—C   *PEC—352*

An example of a parasympatholytic is atropine. A parasympatholytic is a drug that antagonizes the parasympathetic nervous system.

46. ANS—B *PEC—356*

Intradermal drugs are most commonly used for diagnostic testing such as for allergies and TB.

47. ANS—D *PEC—356*

Nitroglycerin patches, some hypertension medications, and hormones are examples of medications given transdermally. A transdermal medication is absorbed through the skin into the circulatory system.

48. ANS—A *PEC—356*

A subcutaneous injection is administered at a 45° angle to the skin.

Figure 13-4

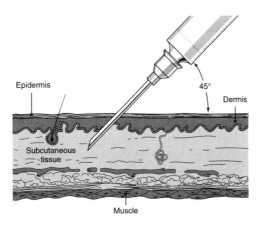

Source: PEC, Figure 13-1F.

49. ANS—B *PEC—356*

An intramuscular injection is administered at a 90° angle to the skin.

Figure 13-5

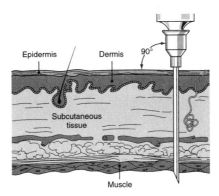

Source: PEC, Figure 13-2F.

50. ANS—D *PEC—356*

It is important to aspirate for blood return when administering medications via the intramuscular route to ensure that the needle is not in a blood vessel.

The conversions are based on the following metric system table:

1 gram = 1000 milligrams = 1,000,000 micrograms
1000 grams = 1 kilogram
1 kilogram = 2.2 pounds
1 liter = 1000 milliliters
1 grain = 60 milligrams

51. ANS—C *PEC—386*

Racemic Epinephrine has both alpha and beta adrenergic receptor stimulation but has a preference for beta-2 thereby causing bronchodilation. It helps relieve the subglottic edema associated with croup.

52. ANS—A *PEC—382*

Procardia (nifedipine) is a calcium channel blocker that is widely used in emergency medicine in the treatment of hypertension. It causes relaxation of the smooth muscles that encircle the peripheral blood vessels resulting in a decrease in diastolic and systolic blood pressure.

53. ANS—D *PEC—388*

Atrovent blocks acetylcholine receptors inhibiting parasympathetic stimulation thereby bronchodilating and drying the respiratory tract.

54. ANS—D *PEC—390*

The oral form of any medication should be deferred in any patient with altered level of consciousness due to possibility of aspiration. D50 should be administered IV only. Glucagon's dose is 0.25–0.5 units and the IM/SQ dose is 1.0 mg. The administration of 1.0 mg Glucagon IM would be the next best step in the management of this patient to start gluconeogenesis. The increase in the patient's blood glucose should make him more cooperative and thus enable an IV to be performed later.

55. ANS—False *PEC—374*

Adenosine should be given as a bolus over 1–2 seconds as its half-life is only 6 seconds. Therefore it should be given in a port that is closest to the patient and flushed with a saline bolus.

56. ANS—False *PEC—376*

Due to its vagolytic effect, Atropine can worsen high AV blocks therefore, it should be avoided and pacing should be implemented.

57. ANS—A *PEC—364*

Dopamine maintains renal and mesenteric perfusion whereas Norepinephrine's alpha effects cause vasoconstriction as does Epinephrine. Dobutamine has no alpha effects but acts primarily on beta-1 receptors in the heart.

58. ANS—B   *PEC—365*

Although Dopamine maintains renal and mesenteric blood flow overall, at doses greater than 20 mcg/kg/min, the alpha-adrenergic receptors predominate causing peripheral vasoconstriction.

59. ANS—B   *PEC—374*

Adenosine is a naturally occurring nucleoside that slows AV conduction through the AV node and interrupts AV reentry pathways in PSVT.

60. ANS—A   *PEC—368*

Due to the adrenergic blockade, beta blockers are contraindicated in asthma/COPD. By blocking the sympathetic receptors, bronchoconstriction will occur—making it harder for the asthmatic to breathe.

61. ANS—A   *PEC—380*

Nitrous oxide is an analgesic/anesthetic gas used for its analgesic properties. The side effects include nausea/vomiting, dizziness, lightheadedness, altered mental status, and hallucinations.

62. ANS—D   *PEC—386*

The beta-2 effects of racemic Epinephrine can cause bronchodilation and is also effective in relieving subglottic edema associated with croup.

63. ANS—B   *PEC—395*

Diphenhydramine is effective in the treatment of dystonic or extrapyramidal reactions as is seen with the phenothiazine drugs.

64. ANS—C   *PEC—368*

Sympathomimetic drugs mimic actions of the sympathetic nervous system and act directly on the receptors or by indirectly stimulating release of catecholamines. All of the above medications are catecholamines except Normodyne (labetolol) which is a beta-blocker.

65. ANS—D   *PEC—372*

Bretylium is an antiarrythmic that exhibits adrenergic and myocardial effects.

66. ANS—D   *PEC—363-6*

The catecholamine group of medications are deactivated by higher pH/alkaline solutions. Therefore, always flush your IV lines when administering epinephrine and sodium bicarbonate.

67. ANS—C   *PEC—369*

Lidocaine (Xylocaine) depresses depolarization, has little effect on atrial tissue and does NOT slow AV conduction nor depress contractility. Lidocaine does increase fibrillation threshold therby acting as a safeguard against the life threatening dysrhythmias.

68. ANS—D   *PEC—369*

Premature ventricular contractions that may lead to life threatening arrhythmias are considered "malignant." All of the above are true except "D" as six is the accepted number.

69. ANS—True   *PEC—370*

Lidocaine slows AV conduction and the decreased ventricular rates associated with high grade heart block can result in escape beats.

70. ANS—False   *PEC—370*

Atropine and external pacing should be utilized first to resolve bradycardia. If the PVC's persist, Lidocaine can be instituted.

71. ANS—A   *PEC—364*

Use of beta blockers with Norepinephrine will exacerbate the alpha effects of the drug and can increase a patient's blood pressure.

72. ANS—C   *PEC—370*

The initial dose of Lidocaine is 1.0–1.5 milligrams per kilogram body weight. It can be repeated every five minutes at 0.5–0.75 mg/kg to a maximum dose of 3 mg/kg.

73. ANS—D   *PEC—374*

Adenocard is metabolized by the red blood cells. It should be administered by rapid IV bolus due to its short half-life.

74. ANS—C   *PEC—376*

Morphine is derived from the opium plant and Digoxin comes from the floxglove plant. Atropine is made from the Atropa belladonna plant group and Adenosine is a natrually occurring nucleoside.

75. ANS—B   *PEC—367-72*

The beta-1 receptor effects when using labetolol causes postural hypotension (p 368). Hypotension is commonly seen following administration of Pronestyl and Bretylol and are indications to use caution and/or discontinue further use of the medications. (p 372). Following Dobutamine administration, tachycardia and hypertension are common (p 367) and can induce or exacerbate myocardial ischemia.

76. ANS—A   *PEC—382*

Procardia causes smooth muscle relaxation primarily in the arterioles thereby decreasing peripheral vascular resistance secondary to peripheral vasodilatation and subsequently decreases systolic and diastolic blood pressure.

77. ANS—B   *PEC—394*

Eclampsia is seen primarily during third trimester pregnancies of first-time mothers. Magnesium sulfate should be started after completion of the ABC's. The standard dose is 2–4 grans IV or IM. Care must be taken to monitor the patient closely for side effects.

Match the following mediation with its action:

78.	dobutamine	**D.**	a positive inotrope, little chronotropy.
79.	dopamine	**B.**	a positive inotrope, a dose-related chronotrope
80.	norepinephrine	**C.**	has alpha and beta effects but more so stimulates alpha receptors
81.	epinephrine	**A.**	has alpha and beta effects but more so stimulates beta receptors

82. ANS—C   *PEC—397*

As long as the airway is patent and being maintained adequately, attempt the use of Narcan/Naloxone to reverse the respiratory depression caused by heroin. The blisters are likely secondary to abscess formation from intravenous injection or the subcutaneous route of administration known as skin popping.

83. ANS—D   *PEC—397*

The standard dose is 1–2 mg that is repeated every 5 minutes. Large doses (i.e. 5–10 mg) may be required for the reversal of synthetics opiates such as Talwin or Darvon.

84. ANS—A   *PEC—397*

Narcan may be administered via all the above methods except orally. If used endotracheally however, it should be diluted in saline and 2–2.5 times the IV dose used.

85. ANS—D   *PEC—394*

Magnesium is indicated during the V-fib algorithm per new ACLS standards and is also indicated for use in preterm labor and/or eclampsia (aka toxemia) associated with gestation.

86. ANS—B   *PEC—393*

Pitocin causes uterine smooth muscles to contract. This stimulates contractions and eventually a delivery of the baby. The contraction also closes the open ended vessels along the endometrium thereby controlling postpartum bleeding. One must be sure that there is only one fetus to be delivered prior to administering this medication.

87. ANS—D   *PEC—394*

Magnesium sulfate is a CNS depressant and also depresses cardiopulmonary function as well. It diminishes deep tendon reflexes also therefore these should be frequently monitored along with the vital signs. If these effects are noted, the infusion should be decreased or discontinued as toxic levels are ensuing.

88. ANS—A   *PEC—395*

Ipecac stimulates vomiting and thus is known as an emetic. It does so by irritating the GI tract and acting on the emetic centers in the brain. Emesis should occur in 5–10 minutes after administration (so be prepared in your small, enclosed, poorly ventilated ambulance for the seemingly long ride that is ahead).

89. ANS—D   *PEC—397*

The dose is 1 gram (1000 mg) charcoal per kilogram weight for children.

90. ANS—B   *PEC—377*

Bicarbonate should not be used early during arrest situations as it has been proven more harmful than good. Once the code has been prolonged and no other intervention is changing the status then it should be considered. Bicarbonate also promotes renal excretion of certain drugs and therefore as an IV infusion, it is used in the management of overdoses. Sodium bicarb is also indicated in the treatment of hyperkalemia to enhance the influx of the potassium ions into the cell.

91. ANS—D   *PEC—378*

The initial dose of bicarbonate is 1 mg/kg followed by repeat dosing of 0.5 mg/kg every ten minutes.

92. ANS—A   *PEC—379*

Nitrous oxide is self administered during cases where analgesia is required such as burns, ischemic pain, fractures, etc. It should be given until the pain is relieved/controlled or the patient drops the mask. This will help to control any overdose potential. The use of the other medications can also be titrated to the patient's pain but are not usually self administered (except in extreme circumstances such as a cancer patient that uses a morphine pump).

93. ANS—D   *PEC—381*

In an emergency the drug should be given IV. The initial dose is 20 mg for patients who do not regularly take the drug and 40–80 mg initially for patients on chronic therapy.

94. ANS—D   *PEC—383*

The calcium channel blockers must be very cautiously used in the face of congestive heart failure as they may preipitate it, especially if the patient is hypotensive. They are also contraindicated in patients receiving beta blockers as bradycardia, asystole, and heart failure may result. The diuretics (such as Lasix/Furosemide) are indicated for their excretion properties. The morphine and nitro are venous vasodilator and help to pool the blood thereby decreasing the workload on the heart; thus are indicated in the treatment of CHF.

95. ANS—C   *PEC—380*

Nitronox tends to diffuse into closed spaces more readily than oxygen or carbon dioxide. Many smokers have weakened pulmonary areas called blebs and the nitrous oxide can concentrate in these areas causing them to swell and rupture, causing a pneumothorax. Nitronox is therefore contraindicated in chest injuries whereby pneumothoraces may be present as the gas will accummulate in the closed space and increase its size.

96. ANS—B   *PEC—382*

Nifedipine is a calcium channel blocker that is used effectively during hypertensive emergencies but it is also effective as a smooth muscle relaxer in the peripheral blood vessels. This in turn decreases peripheral resistance, causes vasodilatation, and decreases systolic and diastolic blood pressure. It is also known to be effective in reducing coronary artery spasm that presents as angina. Cocaine is a vasospastic drug and is known to cause angina that can lead to ischemia and infarction. Angina secondary to coronary vasospasm is termed Prinzmetals Angina.

97. ANS—C   *PEC—383*

Calcium chloride is effective in reducing toxicity associated with magnesium sulfate toxicity.

98. ANS—C   *PEC—383*

Calcium chloride will cause precipitates to form when administered with bicarbonate but this combination along with insulin, is the therapy for hyperkalemia. It can cause all of the side effects as listed in"D" however, it raises digoxin levels and therefore caution must be used to avoid the patients becoming digitalis toxic.

99. ANS—A   *PEC—385*

Aminophylline does relax smooth muscle without affecting adrenergic receptors. It also stimulates the brain's respiratory center. Aminophylline does have some diuretic properties and therefore is useful in treating pulmonary edema nad CHF (not presticide poisioning). This drug is proarrhythmic therefore, it causes arrythmias and caution must be used when a patient is exhibiting hypotension, PVC's, or other arrhythmias. As aminophylline is affected by metabolism in the liver, use with erythromycin can cause toxicity as they both are cleared there.

100. ANS—C   *PEC—382*

The contraindications for nitroglycerin include patients in shock, those who are allergic to it, or those who are hypotensive as this may exacerbate the hypotension. It is also not indicated for use in patients with increased intracranial pressure as the brain may require higher systemic pressures to maintain cerebral blood flow.

101. 1 kilogram = 1000 grams ; 3 kilograms = **3000 grams.**   *PEC—353*

102. 1 gram = 1000 grams ; 2.5 grams = **2500 milligrams**   *PEC—353*

103. 1 milligram = 1000 micrograms ; 8 milligrams = **8000 micrograms**

PEC—353

104. 1000 milliliters = 1 liter ; 3000 milliliters = **3 liters**   *PEC—353*

105. 1 grain = 60 milligrams ; 1/4 grain = **15 milligrams**   *PEC—353*

106. 2.2 lbs. = 1 kilogram ; 22 lbs. = **10 kilograms**   *PEC—353*

107. 1000 micrograms = 1 milligram ; 800 micrograms = **0.8 milligrams**

PEC—353

108. 1 liter = 1000 milliliters ; 3 liters = **3000 milliliters**   *PEC—353*

109. 1000 milligrams = 1 gram ; 500 milligrams = **0.5 grams**   *PEC—353*

110. 1 gram = 1000000 micrograms ; 5 grams = **5000000 micrograms**

PEC—353

111. The patient weighs 176 lbs. 176 ÷ 2.2 = 80 kg   *PEC—355*
1 mg × 80 kg = **80 mg**

112. Patient weighs 220 lbs. 220 ÷ 2.2 = 100 kg   *PEC—355*
10 mg × 100 kg = **1000 mg**

113. Patient weighs 55 lbs. 55 ÷ 2.2 = 25 kg   *PEC—355*
20 ml × 25 kg = **500 ml**

114. Patient weighs 110 lbs. 110 ÷ 2.2 = 50 kg   *PEC—355*
50 kg. × 5 mcg/kg/min = **250 mcg/min**

115. Patient weighs 22 lbs. 22 ÷ 2.2 = 10 kg   *PEC—355*
10 kg × 0.1 mg/kg = **1.0 mg**

116. 100 mg ÷ 10 ml = **10 mg / ml**   *PEC—354*

117. 50 mg ÷ 2 ml = **25 mg/ml**   *PEC—354*

118. 250 mg ÷ 20 ml = **12.5 mg/ml**   *PEC—354*

119. 1 gram (1000 mg) ÷ 10 ml = **100 mg/ml**   *PEC—354*

120. 1 mg ÷ 1 ml = **1 mg/ml**   *PEC—354*

The following calculations are based on the formula:

$$X = \frac{\text{Volume on Hand} \times \text{Desired Dose}}{\text{Drug on hand}}$$

121. $X = \dfrac{5 \text{ ml} \times 75 \text{ mg}}{100 \text{ mg}}$ $\qquad X = \dfrac{375}{100}$ $\qquad$ **X = 3.75 ml**

$\qquad$ *PEC—354*

122. $X = \dfrac{1 \text{ ml} \times 0.25 \text{ mg}}{1 \text{ mg}}$ $\qquad X = \dfrac{0.25}{1}$ $\qquad$ **X = 0.25 ml** $\qquad$ *PEC—354*

123. $X = \dfrac{2 \text{ ml} \times 25 \text{ mg}}{50 \text{ mg}}$ $\qquad X = \dfrac{50}{50}$ $\qquad$ **X = 1 ml** $\qquad$ *PEC—354*

124. $X = \dfrac{5 \text{ ml} \times 50 \text{ mg}}{200 \text{ mg}}$ $\qquad X = \dfrac{250}{200}$ $\qquad$ **X = 1.25 ml** $\qquad$ *PEC—354*

125. $X = \dfrac{10 \text{ ml} \times 0.5 \text{ mg}}{1 \text{ mg}}$ $\qquad X = \dfrac{5.0}{1}$ $\qquad$ **X = 5.0 ml** $\qquad$ *PEC—354*

126. Patient weighs 198 lbs. $198 \div 2.2 = 90$ kg

$\qquad$ MD order is 5 mg/kg $\qquad 90 \text{ kg} \times 5 \text{ mg} = 450 \text{ mg}$

$\qquad X = \dfrac{10 \text{ ml} \times 450 \text{ mg}}{500 \text{ mg}}$ $\qquad X = \dfrac{4500}{500}$ $\qquad$ **X = 9 ml** $\qquad$ *PEC—355*

127. Patient weighs 187 lbs. $187 \div 2.2 = 85$ kg

$\qquad$ MD order is 1 mg/kg $\qquad 85 \text{ kg} \times 1 \text{ mg} = 85 \text{ mg}$

$\qquad X = \dfrac{10 \text{ ml} \times 85 \text{ mg}}{100 \text{ mg}}$ $\qquad X = \dfrac{850}{100}$ $\qquad$ **X = 8.5 ml** $\qquad$ *PEC—355*

128. $X = \dfrac{1 \text{ ml} \times 10 \text{ mg}}{2 \text{ mg}}$ $\qquad X = \dfrac{10}{2}$ $\qquad$ **X = 5 ml** $\qquad$ *PEC—355*

129. $X = \dfrac{10 \text{ ml} \times 120 \text{ mg}}{40 \text{ mg}}$ $\qquad X = \dfrac{1200}{40}$ $\qquad$ **X = 30 ml** $\qquad$ *PEC—355*

130. $X = \dfrac{20 \text{ ml} \times 80 \text{ mg}}{400 \text{ mg}}$ $\qquad X = \dfrac{1600}{400}$ $\qquad$ **X = 4 ml** $\qquad$ *PEC—355*

The following drip rate calculations are based on the formula:

$$X = \frac{\text{Solution volume} \times \text{dose/min} \times \text{Drops/ml in solution set}}{\text{Drug in solution}}$$

131. $X = \dfrac{250 \text{ ml} \times 3 \text{ mg/min} \times 60 \text{ drops/ml}}{1000 \text{ mg}}$ *PEC—355*

$X = \dfrac{750 \times 60}{1000}$ $X = \dfrac{4500}{1000}$ $X = 45$ drops/min

132. $X = \dfrac{500 \text{ ml} \times 2 \text{ mg/min} \times 60 \text{ drops/ml}}{2000 \text{ mg}}$ *PEC—355*

$X = \dfrac{1000 \times 60}{2000}$ $X = \dfrac{60000}{2000}$ $X = 30$ drops/min

133. $X = \dfrac{250 \text{ ml} \times 4 \text{ mcg/min} \times 60 \text{ drops/ml}}{1 \text{ mg } (1000 \text{ mcg})}$ *PEC—355*

$X = \dfrac{1000 \times 60}{2000}$ $X = \dfrac{60000}{2000}$ $X = 60$ drops/min

134. Patient weighs 176 lbs. $176 \div 2.2 = 80$ kg   *PEC—355*
      Md Order is 5 mcg/kg $80 \times 5 = 400$ mcg

$X = \dfrac{500 \text{ ml} \times 400 \text{ mcg} \times 60}{400 \text{ mg } (400000 \text{ mcg})}$

$X = \dfrac{200000 \times 60}{400000}$ $X = \dfrac{12000000}{400000}$ $X = 30$ drops/min

135. $X = \dfrac{500 \text{ ml} \times 2 \text{ mg/min} \times 60 \text{ drops/ml}}{1000 \text{ mg}}$ *PEC—355*

$X = \dfrac{1000 \times 60}{1000}$ $X = \dfrac{60000}{1000}$ $X = 60$ drops/min

DIVISION 3—TRAUMA

CHAPTER 14

Kinetics of Trauma

QUESTIONS

1. Guidelines to aid the prehospital provider in determining which patients require immediate transport to a trauma center are known as
A. mechanism of injury standards
B. injury severity indexes
C. standing orders
D. trauma triage protocols

2. Which of the following mechanisms of injury indicate rapid transport to a trauma center?
A. Falls greater than 20 feet
B. Death of another car occupant
C. Ejection from vehicle
D. All of the above

3. Which of the following physical findings indicate rapid transport to a trauma center?
A. Pulse greater than 100
B. Glasgow coma score greater than 13
C. Femur fracture
D. Airway burns

4. A car traveling at 55 mph will tend to remain traveling at 55 mph until something stops it or slows it down. This is known as the law of
   A. kinetics
   B. inertia
   C. energy
   D. motion

5. Which of the following will generate the greatest amount of kinetic energy?
   A. 20 lb object traveling at 50 mph
   B. 30 lb object traveling at 40 mph
   C. 40 lb object traveling at 30 mph
   D. 50 lb object traveling at 20 mph

6. Axial loading occurs when
   A. the shoulder strikes the side window
   B. the head strikes the front windshield
   C. the knee strikes the lower dashboard
   D. the chest strikes the steering wheel

7. Injuries from the "paper bag syndrome" include
   A. subdural hematoma
   B. pericardial tamponade
   C. lacerated trachea
   D. pneumothorax

8. Which of the following statements is true regarding lateral impact accidents?
   A. The greater amount of passenger protection lessens the injury pattern
   B. They account for the least percentage of vehicular deaths
   C. The amount of vehicular damage exaggerates the injury pattern
   D. None of the above

9. The most commonly seen injury associated with rear-impact accidents is
   A. kidney laceration
   B. lumbar spine fracture
   C. cervical spine injuries
   D. cardiac contusion

10. Which of the following injury patterns are most associated with frontal motorycle accidents in which the driver is ejected?
   A. Lateral pelvis dislocations
   B. Bilateral femur fractures
   C. Spleen and liver lacerations
   D. Crushing injurues

11. Which of the following statements is true regarding pedestrian accidents?
   A. Adults tend to turn away prior to impact
   B. Children tend to face the oncoming car prior to impact
   C. Adults are often thrown up and over the bumper

D. All of the above

12. When assessing falls, you should focus your attention to
A. the height of the fall
B. the surface the victim fell onto
C. the body part that hit first
D. all of the above

13. Primary injuries from a blast include
A. extremity fractures
B. liver lacerations
C. lung injuries
D. impaled objects

14. Secondary injuries from a blast include
A. extremity fractures
B. liver lacerations
C. lung injuries
D. impaled objects

15. Tertiary injuries from a blast include
A. extremity fractures
B. liver lacerations
C. lung injuries
D. impaled objects

16. Which of the following factors will determine a bullet's trajectory?
A. Gravity
B. Wind speed
C. Bullet speed
D. All of the above

17. A bullet's profile refers to its
A. speed
B. trajectory
C. size and shape
D. drag

18. The formation of a partial vacuum within the body from a high-velocity projectile is called
A. profilation
B. cavitation
C. ballistication
D. none of the above

19. Which of the following statements is true regarding knife injuries?
A. Men attackers usually stab downward
B. Women attackers usually stab upward and outward
C. Impaled knives should never be removed in the field
D. None of the above

20. Which of the following penetrating injuries has the greatest energy transfer?
A. Shotgun blast

B. .38 caliber handgun
C. Bow and arrow
D. High speed rifle

ANSWERS

1. ANS—D *PEC—403*

Trauma triage protocols are guidelines that help prehospital personnel determine which patients require immediate transportation to a Trauma Center. They identify the mechanism of injury that can cause serious internal trauma and they establish the physical or clinical findings that reflect serious internal injury.

2. ANS—D *PEC—405*

The following mechanisms of injury indicate rapid transportation to a trauma center:

    Falls greater than 20 feet
    Death of a car occupant
    Struck by a vehicle traveling over 20 mph
    Ejection from the vehicle
    Severe vehicle deformity
    Rollover with signs of impact

3. ANS—D *PEC—405*

The following physical findings indicate rapid transport to a trauma center:

    Pulse greater than 120 or less than 50
    Systolic blood pressure less than 90
    Respiratory rate less than 10 or greater than 29
    Glasgow coma scale less than 13
    Penetrating trauma except for extremities
    Greater than 2 proximal long bone fractures
    Flail chest
    Burns that are greater than 15 percent of body surface area
    Burns to the face or airway

4. ANS—B *PEC—406*

Sir Isaac Newton described the law of inertia. It states that an object at rest tends to remain at rest while an object in motion tends to remain in motion unless acted on by an external force. Therefore, a car traveling a 55 mph will tend to remain traveling at 55 mph until something stops it (i.e., another car, tree, telephone pole, wall) or slows it down (i.e., brakes, road friction, gravity).

5. ANS—A *PEC—406*

Kinetic energy is the energy of motion. It can be measured by the following formula:

$$\frac{\text{Mass (weight)} \times \text{velocity}^2}{2}$$

Using this formula, speed becomes the most important factor. Even the lightest object (20 lbs.) traveling at the fastest speed (50 mph) will generate the greatest amount of kinetic energy.

6. ANS—B *PEC—414*

Axial loading is the application of forces of trauma along the axis of the spine. When the head hits the windshield, that force is transmitted down the cervical spine, often causing compressions of those vertebrae.

7. ANS—D *PEC—414*

The paper bag syndrome is a common injury process associated with steering wheel impact. The driver takes a deep breath in anticipation of the collision. When the chest impacts the steering wheel lung tissue ruptures much like an inflated paper bag caught between clapping hands. Pneumothorax and pulmonary contusion may result.

Figure 14-1

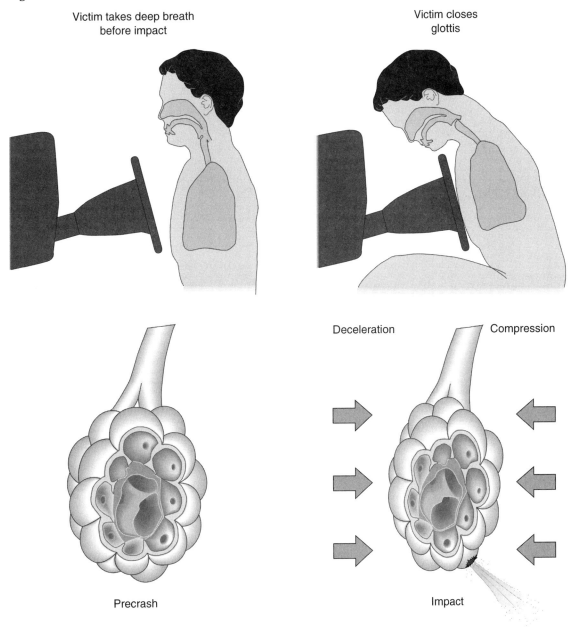

Source: PEC, Figure 14-11.

8. ANS—D   *PEC—414*

Lateral impacts account for 15 percent of all auto accidents yet they are responsible for 22 percent of vehicular fatalities. The amount of structural steel between the impact side and the vehicle interior is greatly reduced. When a lateral impact occurs, the index of suspicion for serious internal injuries should be higher than vehicle damage alone suggests.

9. ANS—C   *PEC—416*

In rear end impact the collision force pushes the auto forward while the vehicle seat propells the occupant forward. If the headrest is not up, the head is unsupported and remains stationary. The neck extends severely while the head rotates backwards. Cervical spine injuries are common with rear-end collisions.

Figure 14-2

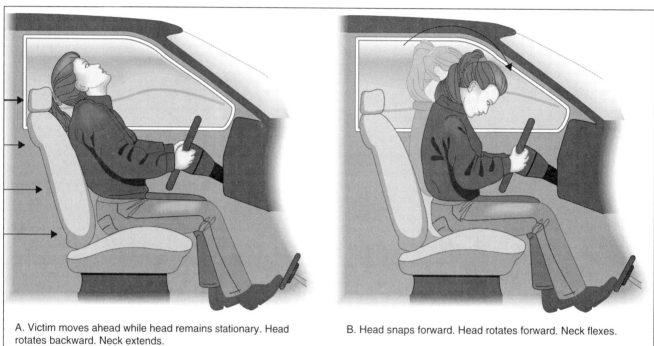

A. Victim moves ahead while head remains stationary. Head rotates backward. Neck extends.

B. Head snaps forward. Head rotates forward. Neck flexes.

Source: PEC, Figure 14-15.

10. ANS—B   *PEC—420*

In frontal or head-on motorcycle accidents, the impact often propells the rider upward and forward. Occasionally the rider traps both femurs at the handlebars causing bilateral fractures.

11. ANS—B   *PEC—420*

In contrast to adults, children turn toward an oncoming vehicle. Because they are smaller the injury is located anatomically higher as the bumper fractures the femur or pelvis.

12. ANS—D   *PEC—422*

When assessing the mechanism of injury of falls, you should evaluate the following aspects: the height of the fall, the landing surface, and the part of the body that impacted first.

13. ANS—C *PEC—424*

Primary blast injuries are caused by the initial air blast and pressure wave. Injuries resulting from the compression of hollow organs such as the lungs include pneumothorax and alveolar rupture.

14. ANS—D *PEC—424*

Secondary blast injuries are caused by flying debris propelled by the force of the blast. Impacting debris may produce blunt or penetrating trauma.

15. ANS—A *PEC—424*

Tertiary blast injuries propel the victim away from the blast and into objects or the ground. Injuries are similar to those found in auto ejection.

16. ANS—D *PEC—426*

A bullet's trajectory refers to the path it follows. This path is modified by a variety of forces. The faster the bullet, the flatter its curve of travel and the straighter its trajectory. As the bullet travels through the air, however, it is constantly pulled down by gravity. As the bullet speed slows its trajectory will become more arched.

17. ANS—C *PEC—426*

A bullet's profile refers to its size and shape as it contacts a target. The larger the diameter of the projectile, or its profile, the more tissue it can contact and the more rapidly it exchanges energy.

18. ANS—B *PEC—426*

Cavitation refers to the formation of a partial vacuum and subsequent cavity within a liquid. This describes the action of a high velocity projectile on the human body which is 60% water. As the bullet passes through body tissue, it causes a wave of pressure to move in front of and along side the projectile leaving the cavity in its wake. This wave compresses organs and tissue causing contusion, rupture, and fracture.

Figure 14-3

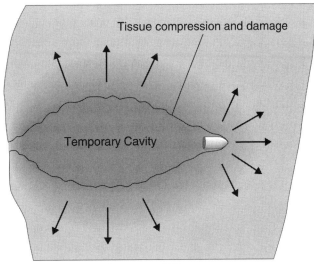

Cavitational Wave

Source: PEC, Figure 14-27.

19. ANS—D   *PEC—428*

Knife-wielding males usually strike with a forward, outward, or crosswise stroke. Females usually strike with an overhand and downward blow. If a knife lodges in the body, it may be dangerous to remove. The only impaled objects that you should remove on the scene are those logged in the cheek and may interfere with the airway or those that you must remove to provide CPR.

20. ANS—D   *PEC—429*

According to Newton's kinetic energy formula, the greater the speed, the greater the energy transfer. A high speed rifle will provide greater kinetic energy because of its greater speed.

CHAPTER 15

Head, Neck, and Spinal Trauma

QUESTIONS

1. The brain and spinal cord make up the
   A. autonomic nervous system
   B. peripheral nervous system
   C. central nervous system
   D. none of the above

2. The three meningeal layers of the brain from the inside-out are the
   A. dura mater, pia mater, arachnoid membrane
   B. pia mater, dura mater, arachnoid membrane
   C. arachnoid membrane, pia mater, dura mater
   D. pia mater, arachnoid membrane, dura mater

3. The prominent bone of the cheek is known as the
   A. mandible
   B. maxilla
   C. sphenoid
   D. zygoma

4. The finger-like process of the second vertebra around which the first cervical vertebra rotates is the
   A. atlas
   B. axis
   C. odontoid
   D. mastoid

5. The opening on the vertebrae through which the spinal cord passes is the
   A. foramen magnum
   B. odontoid process
   C. spinal foramen
   D. dura mater

6. Cerebrospinal fluid circulates through which meningeal layer?
   A. Epidural space
   B. Subdural space
   C. Subarachnoid space
   D. Intracerebral space

7. Central nervous system neurons cannot regenerate after injury because they lack the protective protein sheath known as the
   A. pia mater
   B. neurilemma
   C. falx cerebri
   D. periosteum

8. The area of the brain that is the center of conscious thought is the
   A. cerebrum
   B. cerebellum
   C. central sulcus
   D. falx cerebri

9. The cerebrum is separated from the cerebellum by the
   A. falx cerebri
   B. central sulcus
   C. cribriform plate
   D. tentorium

10. The irregular bone at the base of the skull is the
   A. falx cerebri
   B. central sulcus
   C. cribriform plate
   D. tentorium

11. The pulse rate, respiration, and blood pressure are controlled in the
   A. pons
   B. falx cerebri
   C. medulla oblongata
   D. cerebellum

12. Topographical regions of the body innervated by specific nerve roots are known as
   A. dermatomes
   B. cauda equina
   C. neurilemma
   D. axons

Match the following parts of the eye with their respective definitions:

13. _____ Vitreous humor **A.** Provides nourishment and lubrication

14. _____ Aqueous humor **B.** Colored portion of the eye

15. _____ Pupil **C.** White, vascular area of the eye

16. _____ Iris **D.** Gelatinous fluid found in eye globe

17. _____ Conjunctiva **E.** Thin, clear layer covering iris and cornea

18. _____ Lacrimal ducts **F.** Liquid found in anterior chamber of eye

19. _____ Sclera **G.** Opening in the center of the iris

20. We hear because of the vibration of the
   A. tympanic membrane
   B. cochlea
   C. semicircular canals
   D. dens

21. Positional sense is regulated by our
   A. tympannic membrane
   B. cochlea
   C. semicircular canals
   D. dens

22. Which of the following statements is true regarding scalp lacerations?
   A. They tend to bleed profusely.
   B. Severe bleeding can lead to shock.
   C. The blood vessels lack muscular control.
   D. All of the above.

23. Battle's sign and periorbital ecchymosis are classic signs of a/an
   A. intracerebral hemorrhage
   B. basilar skull fracture
   C. depressed skull fracture
   D. subdural hematoma

24. A brain injury occurring on the opposite side of the impact is known as a
   A. concussion
   B. contusion
   C. contrecoup
   D. cochlea

25. A patient who has sustained a closed head injury with a brief loss of consciousness but no tissue damage and a complete recovery of function has suffered a
   A. concussion
   B. contusion
   C. contrecoup
   D. cochlea

26. A patient who has sustained a closed head injury with resulting tissue damage has suffered a
   A. concussion
   B. contusion
   C. contrecoup
   D. cochlea

27. A pool of blood in the anterior chamber of the eye is known as
   A. conjunctival hemorrhage
   B. retinal artery occlusion
   C. hyphema
   D. corneal abrasion

28. A patient who compains of sudden painless loss of vision in one eye has most likely suffered a
   A. retinal detachment
   B. retinal artery occlusion
   C. hyphema
   D. blowout fracture

29. Subcutaneous emphysema in the neck region is normally caused by
   A. jugular vein laceration
   B. carotid artery laceration
   C. laryngo-tracheal laceration
   D. cervical spine injury

30. Which of the following is a complication of jugular vein laceration?
   A. Pulmonary embolism
   B. Air embolism
   C. Hemorrhagic shock
   D. All of the above

31. Which of the following is **NOT** part of "Cushing's Response?"
   A. Hypertension
   B. Bradycardia
   C. Altered respirations
   D. Hypothermia

32. A patient who responds only to deep pain by abnormally flexing the arms has a Glasgow Coma Score of
   A. 3
   B. 5
   C. 7
   D. 9

SCENARIO   Your patient is a 75-year-old nursing home resident who presents with a decreased level of response. The staff claims he began acting strangely hours before calling you. He has no history of diabetes or CNS disease. His only history is that of a minor fall he took one week ago. He presents with a slow bounding pulse, systolic blood pressure of 170, which is high for him, an erratic breathing pattern and a slightly larger right pupil. His blood sugar is 120, and there is no history or evidence of substance abuse.

33. This patient has probably suffered a/an
A. epidural hematoma
B. subdural hematoma
C. basilar skull fracture
D. concussion

34. The signs and symptoms of this type of injury often present themselves hours or days following the injury because
A. significant brain swelling takes that long to develop
B. the bleeding is from a small vein
C. the bleeding is from a large artery
D. there is no real tissue damage

35. High risk factors for this type of injury include
A. alcoholism
B. the elderly
C. recent head injuries
D. all of the above

SCENARIO Your patient is a 25-year-old boxer who was knocked out with a left hook to the side of the head and now lies in the dressing room fully awake. His initial vital signs are: BP—130 / 80, pulse 80, respirations 18, pupils equal and reactive to light. Enroute to the hospital, he begins to lose consciousness and complains of being sleepy. His breathing becomes erratic, his pulse slows to 60, and his blood pressure rises to 180/90. His left pupil is larger than the right and is slow to react to light.

36. This patient is probably suffering from a/an
A. epidural hematoma
B. subdural hematoma
C. basilar skull fracture
D. concussion

37. The rapid onset of signs and symptoms is most likely due to the
A. fracture of the cribiform plate
B. rupture of the middle meningeal artery
C. leakage of CSF into soft tissues
D. jarring of the reticular activating system

38. This patient also shows the classic signs and symptoms of
A. increasing intracranial pressure
B. decreasing cerebral blood volume
C. basilar skull fracture
D. contracoup injury

39. These signs and symptoms are caused by
A. brain shrinkage
B. cerebral blood flow interruption
C. brainstem herniation
D. abnormally low carbon dioxide levels

40. His abnormal breathing pattern is caused by
A. high levels of carbon dioxide

    B. pressure on the medulla

    C. the leakage of cerebrospinal fluid into the nasal cavity

    D. foramen magnum collapse

41. This patient may hyperventilate in an attempt to

    A. vasodilate the brain vasculature

    B. vasoconstrict the brain vasculature

    C. increase carbon dioxide levels

    D. cause a metabolic alkalosis

42. The larger left pupil is caused by compression of the

    A. third cranial nerve

    B. reticular activating system

    C. extraoccular muscles

    D. iris muscle

43. This patient may vomit without accompanying nausea due to

    A. high levels of carbon dioxide

    B. brain hypoxia

    C. Cushing's reflex

    D. pressure on the medulla

44. Prehospital management of this patient includes all of the following **EXCEPT**

    A. hyperventilation with 100% oxygen

    B. intubation

    C. spinal immobilization

    D. care should include all of the above

45. Pharmacological therapy for this patient may include

    A. furosemide

    B. methylprednisolone

    C. Solu-Medrol

    D. all of the above

SCENARIO Your patient is a 45-year-old male who was ejected from a vehicle in a one-car rollover accident. He presents on the ground complaining of the inability to move his arms and legs. His airway is clear and his vital signs are: respirations 18 with no chest rise, BP—70/30, pulse 60, skin warm and dry. He also presents with priapism and the hands in the "hold-up" position.

46. Your field diagnosis of this patient should include

    A. neurogenic shock

    B. cervical spinal cord interruption

    C. bilateral paralysis

    D. all of the above

47. His unusual vital sign presentation is due to

    A. peripheral nerve interruption

    B. loss of sympathetic nervous system control

    C. loss of parasympathetic nervous system control

    D. blood loss below the injury

48. The priapism is caused by
   A. parasympathetic stimulation
   B. sympathetic stimulation
   C. total autonomic nervous system dysfunction
   D. none of the above

49. The absence of chest rise is due to
   A. intercostal muscle paralysis
   B. rupture of the diaphragm
   C. damage to the third cranial nerve
   D. Cushing's reflex

50. Prehospital management includes which of the following procedures?
   A. IV fluid replacement
   B. Pneumatic antishock garment
   C. Spinal immobilization
   D. All of the above

DRUG REVIEW

Drug	Adult	Pediatric
Furosemide		
Methylprednisolone		
Diazepam		

ANSWERS

1. ANS—C   *PEC—435*

The central nervous system consists of the brain and spinal cord. It regulates all voluntary and involuntary body functions, maintains consciousness, and permits our awareness of the environment.

2. ANS—D   *PEC—438*

The meninges is a group of three tissues between the skull and the brain and between the inside of the spinal foramen and the cord. The outermost layer is the dura mater. The layer closest to the brain and spinal cord is the pia mater and separating the two layers is connective tissue called the arachnoid membrane. From the inside-out, they form a "PAD" for the brain and spinal cord.

3. ANS—D   *PEC—435*

The zygoma is the prominent bone of the cheek. It protects the eyes and the muscles controlling eye and jaw movement.

4. ANS—C   *PEC—436*

The second cervical vertebrae, the axis, has a small finger-like upper projection, called the odontoid process, that forms the pivot point around which the head rotates. The first cervical vertebrae, the atlas, sits atop this protrusion.

5. ANS—C   *PEC—438*

The spinal foramen is the opening in the vertebrae through which the spinal cord passes. The cord travels from the skull to the second lumbar vertebrae. This tube must remain alligned to prevent injury to the spinal cord.

6. ANS—C   *PEC—439*

Beneath the arachnoid membrane is the subarachnoid space which is filled with cerebrospinal fluid. Cerebrospinal fluid is the medium that surrounds the central nervous system and acts to absorb the shock of minor deceleration.

7. ANS—B *PEC—439*

Central nervous system neurons differ in structure from peripheral neurons. They do not have the protective protein sheet called neurilemma along their long axon. This subtle difference is important when considering trauma and regenerative repair. When injured, peripheral nerves may regenerate along the pathway provided by the neurilemma. In the central nervous system, however, injury that either interrupts the axon or kills the cell is generally permanent.

8. ANS—A *PEC—439*

The cerebrum is the largest of the brain regions and occupies most of the cranial cavity. It is the center of conscious thought, personality, speech, motor control, and visual, auditory, and tactile perception.

9. ANS—D *PEC—440*

The tentorium is an extension of the dura mater separating the cerebrum from the cerebellum. It is a fibrous sheet and runs at right angles to the falx cerebri.

10. ANS—C *PEC—440*

The cribriform plate is an irregular and bony plane at the base of the skull. It has surfaces against which the brain may abrade, lacerate, or contuse in severe deceleration injuries. This is the location of the common basilar skull fracture.

11. ANS—C *PEC—440*

The medulla oblongata is a bulge in the very top of the spinal cord. It controls pulse rate, respiration, and blood pressure. Located just above the foramen magnum this structure is often affected by a rise in intracranial pressure.

Figure 15-1

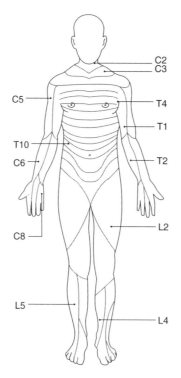

Source: PEC, Figure 15-4.

12. ANS—A *PEC—440*

Dermatomes are body regions corresponding to various nerve routes. As these peripheral routes branch off the spine they perceive sensation lower and lower on the body.

13. _____	Vitreous humor	**D.** Gelatinous fluid found in eye globe
14. _____	Aqueous humor	**F.** Liquid found in anterior chamber of eye
15. _____	Pupil	**G.** Opening in the center of the iris
16. _____	Iris	**B.** Colored portion of the eye
17. _____	Conjunctiva	**E.** Thin, clear layer covering iris and cornea
18. _____	Lacrimal ducts	**A.** Provides nourishment and lubrication
19. _____	Sclera	**C.** White, vascular area of the eye

20. ANS—A *PEC—443*

Hearing occurs when sound waves cause the tympanic membrane, or ear drum, to vibrate. The ear drum transmits the vibrations through three very small bones to the cochlea, the organ of hearing. These vibrations stimulate the auditory nerve which in turn transmits the signal to the brain.

21. ANS—C *PEC—443*

The semicircular canals are three rings of the inner ear. They are responsible for sensing the motion of the head and providing positional sense for the body. This positional sense is present even when the eyes are closed. If injury or illness disturbs this center, excess signals are sent to the brain. Patients complain of a spinning feeling known as vertigo.

22. ANS—D *PEC—444*

The scalp is an area frequently subjected to soft tissue injury. Because this area is extremely vascular and because the scalp vessels are larger and not quite as muscular as other vessels, blood loss can be rapid and difficult to control. Severe and persistent bleeding from scalp lacerations can contribute to shock.

23. ANS—B *PEC—445*

Battle's sign is a black and blue discoloration over the mastoid process just behind the ear. Bilateral periorbital ecchymosis is a black and blue discoloration of the area surrounding the eyes. Both of these signs are normally associated with a basular skull fracture.

24. ANS—C *PEC—448*

A contracoup injury occurs on the opposite side of the side of impact. The brain impacts the interior of the skull on the opposite side causing soft tissue injury such as contusions, lacerations, and hemorrages.

25. ANS—A *PEC—448*

A person who has sustained a closed head injury with a brief loss of consciousness but no tissue damage and a complete recovery of function, has suffered a concussion.

26. ANS—B *PEC—448*

A contusion is a more significant jarring than a concussion and results in cell damage. It is a closed wound in which the skin is unbroken, although damage has occurred to the tissue beneath. If the loss of consciousness is longer than five minutes the patient is usually admitted to the hospital.

27. ANS—C   *PEC—452*

Hemorrhage into the anterior chamber of the eye will pool and display a level of blood in front of the pupil and iris. This condition is known as hyphema and is not emergent. It does, however, require evaluation by an opthamologist.

28. ANS—B   *PEC—453*

Retinal artery occlusion is a vascular emergency in which an embolus, or traveling clot, blocks the blood supply to the eye. The patient complains of sudden and painless loss of vision in one eye.

29. ANS—C   *PEC—453*

Penetrating wounds or tears to the trachea or larynx may force air into the neck during expiration. Upon assessment you may feel a crackling sensation called subcutaneous emphysema or notice a gradual increase in the diameter of the neck.

30. ANS—D   *PEC—453*

Jugular veins at times maintain a pressure less than atmospheric. An open wound may draw air into a vessel affecting the heart or pulmonary circulation. Jugular veins, although rather low-pressure vessels, still carry large volumes of blood and will bleed profusely.

31. ANS—D   *PEC—450*

In cases of increasing intracranial pressure, the brain displaces away from the side of the hematoma toward the foramen magnum. This movement pushes the medulla oblongata into the foramen magnum producing changes in vital signs. The pulse rate slows, respirations become erratic, and the blood pressure rises. This collective change in vital signs is called "Cushing's Response."

Figure 15-2

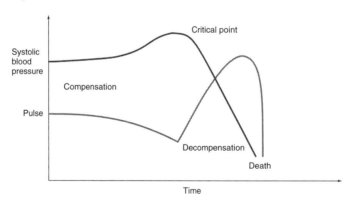

Source: PEC, Figure 15-15.

32. ANS—B   *PEC—459*

The Glascow Coma Scale objectively rates your patient in three categories: eye opening, best motor response, and best verbal response. Since this patient does not open his eyes, he gets a score of one in the first category. Since he does not respond to verbal commands, he gets a one in the second category. He flexes abnormally to pain, earning a score of three in the last category, making his total score five.

33. ANS—B   *PEC—449*

A subdural hematoma is a collection of blood directly beneath the dura mater.

34. ANS—B *PEC—449*

The signs and symptoms following a subdural hematoma occur very slowly and are subtle in presentation because blood loss is usually due to rupture of a small venous vessel.

35. ANS—D *PEC—449*

You will frequently encounter subdural hematomas in elderly patients or chronic alcoholics. Because the aging process and chronic alcoholism shrink the brain, both groups are prone to this condition following even seemingly minor head injuries. Your patient's altered behavior pattern may be caused by a subdural hematoma.

36. ANS—A *PEC—449*

Epidural hematoma is an accumulation of blood between the dura mater and the cranium.

37. ANS—B *PEC—450*

The rapid onset of signs and symptoms following an epidural hematoma occurs because the bleeding involves arterial vessels, often the middle meningeal artery. The condition progresses rapidly while the patient moves quickly toward unconsciouness. Since the bleeding is arterial, intracranial pressure builds rapidly compressing the cerebrum and increasing the pressure within the skull.

38. ANS—A *PEC—450*

This patient shows the classic signs and symptoms of increasing intracranial pressure: an altered respiratory pattern, bradycardia, hypertension, unequal pupils, and a decreasing level of consciousness.

39. ANS—C *PEC—450*

These signs and symptoms are caused by brain herniation. As the pressure in the cranium increases, the brain is pushed downward through the tentorium toward the brainstem. Because the brainstem houses our cardiac and respiratory centers, these vital signs are affected.

40. ANS—B *PEC—450*

Pressure on the medulla oblongata causes alterations in respiratory control. Your patient may hyperventilate, exhibit Cheyne-Stokes respirations, and eventually stop breathing altogether.

41. ANS—B *PEC—450*

High levels of carbon dioxide cause the brain vasculature to dilate. This results in increased blood volume which in turn increases the pressure within the skull. In an attempt to vasoconstrict these vessels and reverse the process, the body may begin to hyperventilate.

42. ANS—A *PEC—450*

Pressure on the third cranial nerve, the occulomotor nerve, causes the pupil on that side to dilate. An early indicator of increasing intracranial pressure is a slightly larger pupil that reacts slowly to light. As the pressure increases, the pupil will become fixed and totally dilated.

43. ANS—D *PEC—450*

The vomit center is located in the medulla oblongata. Pressure on this center will cause immediate vomiting without accompanying nausea. The vomiting is usually forceful and known as "projectile vomiting."

44. ANS—D *PEC—460*

Prehospital management of a patient with increasing intracranial pressure includes the following: spinal immobilization; aggressive airway management and intubation as soon as possible to protect the airway from the eventual vomiting; high flow O2 to maximize brain oxygenation and prevent tissue swelling; and hyperventilation with a bag-valve-mask at a rate of 24/minute to vasoconstrict the brain.

45. ANS—D *PEC—466*

Pharmacological therapy for this patient may include a diuretic such as furosemide to decrease intravascular blood volume; a steroid such as methylprednisolone to decrease tissue swelling; or an anticonvulsant such as diazepam to control seizures.

46. ANS—D *PEC—452*

Your prehospital diagnosis of this patient should include cervical spinal cord interruption, bilateral paralysis and neurogenic shock.

47. ANS—B *PEC—452*

Patients in shock usually present with hypotension, tachycardia, and cool, clammy skin. These signs indicate that the sympathetic nervous system compensatory mechanism has been activated. Your patient's unusual vital sign presentation (i.e., hypotension, bradycardia, warm and dry skin) indicates the loss of sympathetic nervous system control.

48. ANS—A *PEC—452*

Priapism is a painful penile erection. In this case it is caused by the loss of sympathetic nervous system tone allowing parasympathetic stimulation to dominate.

49. ANS—A *PEC—452*

Interruption of the spinal cord in the cervical region will cause the intercostal muscles of the chest to become dysfunctional. Patients with this problem exhibit "belly breathing" characterized by movement of the diaphragm.

50. ANS—D *PEC—462*

Prehospital management of this patient includes spinal immobilization, pneumatic anti-shock garment, and IV fluid replacement with normal saline or Lactated Ringer's.

DRUG REVIEW

Drug	Adult	Pediatric
Furosemide	20—80 mg IV	
Methylprednisolone	30 mg / kg IV	
Diazepam	2—15 mg IV	

CHAPTER 16

Body Cavity Trauma

QUESTIONS

1. The central cavity within the thorax that houses the major chest organs is the
   A. central sulcus
   B. manubrium
   C. peritoneum
   D. mediastinum

2. The uppermost part of the sternum is the
   A. mediastinum
   B. manubrium
   C. sternal body
   D. xiphoid process

3. The heart is suspended in the chest by the aortic arch and the ligamentum
   A. arteriosum
   B. cardiosum
   C. teres
   D. pericardium

4. The kidneys, spleen, and part of the pancreas are located within the _____ cavity.
   A. peritoneal
   B. retroperitoneal

    C. pleural

    D. pericardial

5. The sigmoid colon is located in the
  A. right upper quadrant
  B. left upper quadrant
  C. right lower quadrant
  D. left lower quadrant

6. The appendix is located in the
  A. right upper quadrant
  B. left upper quadrant
  C. right lower quadrant
  D. left lower quadrant

7. The gallbladder is located in the
  A. right upper quadrant
  B. left upper quadrant
  C. right lower quadrant
  D. left lower quadrant

8. The stomach is located in the
  A. right upper quadrant
  B. left upper quadrant
  C. right lower quadrant
  D. left lower quadrant

9. The continuous tube that extends from the esophagus to the rectum is the _____ canal.
  A. duodenal
  B. alimentary
  C. parenteral
  D. peritoneal

10. The wave-like muscular motion of the intestines is known as
  A. alimentation
  B. paristalsis
  C. omentum
  D. mesentary action

11. Which of the following is a function of the liver?
  A. Detoxifying blood from the intestines
  B. Storing body energy reserves
  C. Producing plasma protiens
  D. All of the above

12. Bile is stored in the
  A. liver
  B. gallbladder
  C. pancreas
  D. spleen

13. The small bowel consists of which following three sections in order?
   A. Ileum, duodenum, jejunum
   B. Jejunum, omentum, duodenum
   C. Duodenum, jejunum, ileum
   D. Omentum, ileum, jejunum

14. A collapse of alveoli is known as
   A. consolidation
   B. atelectasis
   C. excursion
   D. effusion

15. The liver is suspended in the abdomen by the
   A. ligamentum teres
   B. bundle of Kent
   C. isle of Langerhans
   D. mesentary

SCENARIO Your patient is a 45-year-old who presents with a bluish discoloration above the nipple line, absent vital signs, bloodshot eyes, and distended neck veins. He was pinned for a short time underneath his car following a rollover accident.

16. He has most likely suffered a
   A. tension pneumothorax
   B. traumatic asphyxia
   C. massive hemothorax
   D. pericardial tamponade

17. The bluish discoloration is caused by
   A. lack of oxygen in the tissues
   B. low PaO_2
   C. the bursting of capillaries
   D. high $PaCO_2$

SCENARIO Your patient is a 35-year-old female who was stabbed in the right chest after a quarrel with her girlfriend. You quickly discover a sucking wound in the right chest. She presents with diminished breath sounds right side, hyperressonant to percussion on right side, ecchymosis from T-5 to T-8 on right side, and dyspnea. BP—120/70, HR 90, RR—26 and shallow.

18. In addition to the sucking wound, your field diagnosis is
   A. massive hemothorax
   B. pneumothorax
   C. pericardial tamponade
   D. tension pneumothorax

19. Her condition is due to
  A. blood in the pleural space
  B. air in the pleural space
  C. blood in the pericardial sac
  D. air in the pericardial sac

20. Your initial management of this patient is to
  A. intubate the trachea
  B. ventilate with 100% oxygen
  C. seal the open wound with an occlusive dressing
  D. decompress the chest immediately

SCENARIO   Your patient is a 15-year-old male who fell off his bicycle and hit the ground very hard. He presents with parodoxical chest movement on the right side, dyspnea, and guarded respirations. His vital signs are: BP—140/80, HR—100, RR—30 and shallow, diminished breath sounds on both sides.

21. Your field diagnosis is
  A. pneumothorax
  B. flail chest
  C. traumatic asphyxia
  D. hemothorax

22. The paradoxical movement is due to
  A. the instability of the chest wall
  B. air in the pleural space
  C. blood in the pleural space
  D. paralysis of the respiratory muscles

23. The major complication from this injury is
  A. bleeding into the pericardial space
  B. air leaking into the subcutaneous tissues
  C. decreased tidal volumes
  D. rib displacement

24. Prehospital management of this patient includes
  A. positive pressure ventilation
  B. emergency chest decompression
  C. pericardiocentesis
  D. having the patient breathe into a paper bag

SCENARIO   Your patient is a 26-year-old who was shot with a small caliber handgun in the right chest. She presents with dyspnea, distended neck veins, absent breath sounds on the right side, diminished breath sounds on the left, hyperressonant on both sides, tracheal deviation toward the left side. Her vital signs are: BP—70/30, pulse 120 and weak, respirations 30 and shallow.

25. Your field diagnosis is
  A. simple pneumothorax

      B. tension pneumothorax
      C. pericardial tamponade
      D. massive hemothorax

26. Her hypotension could be caused by
      A. decreased venous return
      B. tamponade effect on the heart
      C. blood loss
      D. all of the above

27. Emergency field management of this patient includes
      A. pneumatic antishock garment
      B. needle chest decompression
      C. pericardiocentesis
      D. none of the above

SCENARIO Your patient is a 67-year-old female who was struck by a car and lies on the ground. She presents with dyspnea, pain to the right chest, dull percussion on the right side, diminished breath sounds on the right side. Her vital signs are: BP—80/60, HR—110, RR—30, skin cool and clammy, flat neck veins.

28. Your field diagnosis is
      A. tension pneumothorax
      B. hemothorax
      C. pericardial tamponade
      D. traumatic asphyxia

29. Emergency field management of this patient includes
      A. rapid IV fluid replacement
      B. pericardiocentesis
      C. needle decompression
      D. pneumatic antishock garment

SCENARIO Your patient is a 35-year-old unbelted male driver who hit the steering wheel and windshield in a one-car accident. He presents unconscious with the following vital signs: BP—110/90, pulse 120 and weak, respirations 28 and shallow, lungs equal and clear, distant heart sounds, skin cool and clammy, and distended neck veins. His only external signs of trauma is a midsternal bruise.

30. Your field diagnosis is
      A. tension pneumothorax
      B. massive hemothorax
      C. traumatic asphyxia
      D. pericardial tamponade

31. This patients primary problem is
      A. air filling the pleural space
      B. fluid in the pericardial sac

     C. severe crushing injury to the chest
     D. blood in the pleural space

32. Emergency management of this patient includes
     A. needle decompression
     B. chest tube
     C. pneumatic antishock garment
     D. pericardiocentesis

SCENARIO Your patient is a 57-year-old female who was a passenger in a two-car accident. She was ejected from the vehicle and lies on the ground next to the car. She presents unconscious with no obvious signs of trauma. Her vital signs are: BP—70/30, pulse 120 and weak, respirations 38 and shallow, lungs equal and clear, flat neck veins. Upon exam, you find discoloration around the umbilicus and abdominal guarding.

33. Your field diagnosis is
     A. tension pneumothorax
     B. pericardial tamponade
     C. intra-abdominal hemorrhage
     D. ruptured diaphragm

34. Abdominal guarding usually indicates
     A. diaphragmatic tear
     B. hypovolemic shock
     C. peritoneal irritation
     D. aortic aneurysm

35. Field management of this patient includes
     A. pneumatic antishock garment
     B. IV fluid replacement
     C. rapid transport to a trauma center
     D. all of the above

ANSWERS **1. ANS—D**   *PEC—472*

The central region of the chest is the mediastinum. It houses several vital structures: the heart, trachea, vena cava, aorta, and esophagus. Each structure is a major conduit for the respiratory, venous, arterial, and digestive systems.

2. ANS—B   *PEC—471*

The sternum is divided into three parts. The uppermost part is a triangular-shaped bone called the manubrium. The manubrium is the attaching point for the clavicles and first ribs.

3. ANS—A   *PEC—473*

The arch of the aorta and the ligamentum arteriosum suspend the heart centrally in the chest. In deceleration accidents, this point of attachment often tears the aorta causing rapid exsanguination and death.

4. ANS—B *PEC—474*

The retroperitoneal space lies behind the layers of the peritoneum. The organs within this space include the kidneys, spleen, and part of the pancreas.

5. ANS—D *PEC—474*

The left lower quadrant houses the sigmoid colon as well as portions of the small and large intestine.

6. ANS—C *PEC—474*

The right lower quadrant contains the appendix.

7. ANS—A *PEC—474*

The right upper quadrant contains the liver, right kidney, gallbladder, duodenum, and part of the pancreas.

8. ANS—B *PEC—474*

The left upper quadrant includes the stomach, left kidney, spleen, and most of the pancreas.

9. ANS—B *PEC—474*

The alimentary canal is a continuous tube that begins with the esophagus and ends with the rectum. In this canal, food goes through the digestive process.

10. ANS—B *PEC—474*

Paristalsis is the wave-like muscular motion of the esophagus and bowel moving food through the digestive system.

11. ANS—D *PEC—474*

The liver occupies the area below and under the ribcage in the right upper quadrant. A large and vascular organ, it detoxifies the blood coming from the digestive field, stores body energy reserves, produces plasma proteins, and performs many other important functions.

12. ANS—B *PEC—474*

Beneath and behind the liver is the gallbladder, a storehouse for bile. Bile is a product of the liver that helps in the digestion of fat.

13. ANS—C *PEC—474*

The small intestine consists of three sections. The first section is called the duodenum. The second section is called the jejunum, and the third section is the ilium.

14. ANS—B *PEC—476*

Shallow breathing results in alveolar collapse. The natural reflex to correct this, the sigh, is suppressed by the pain. This alveolar collapse is called atelectasis and results in less efficient respiration and over the long term may lead to pneumonia or other respiratory infection.

15. ANS—A *PEC—482*

The ligamentum teres suspends the liver. In deceleration the ligament may slice the liver as cheese is sliced by a wire cutter. This laceration is severe often resulting in rapid hemorrhage.

16. ANS—B *PEC—476*

Sudden compression of the chest from a crushing injury can lead to traumatic asphyxia. The compression severely limits chest excursion and results in hypoventilation. It may also cause a backup of venous blood within the head and neck causing the classic bloodshot eyes, bulging blue tongue, distended neck veins, and cyanotic upper body, the classic "hood sign."

17. ANS—C   *PEC—477*

Backflow of venous blood through the jugular veins into the head causes tremendous pressures in the capillaries resulting in bursting. The result is petechiae which gives the patient a purplish look above the nipples.

18. ANS—B   *PEC—478*

This patient's presentation of diminished breath sounds on the right side with hyperresonance and ecchymosis all indicate pneumothorax.

19. ANS—B   *PEC—478*

A pneumothorax is caused by a tear in the pleura. Air enters the pleural space collapsing the lung in that particular area.

Figure 16-1

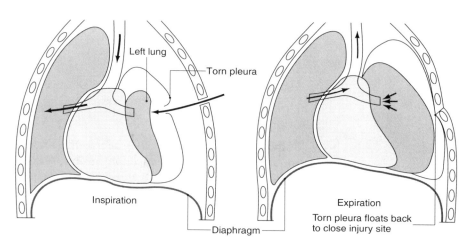

Source: PEC, Figure 16-12.

20. ANS—C   *PEC—478*

Initial management of this patient is aimed at sealing the wound with an occlusive dressing during exhalation. At the end of exhalation, cover the wound and tape it on three sides to prevent air from entering upon inhalation, but allowing air to escape during exhalation.

21. ANS—B   *PEC—476*

Paradoxical chest movement is a classic sign of a flail chest. Flail chest occurs when three or more ribs are fractured in multiple places causing a floating segment reducing the stability of the chest wall.

22. ANS—A   *PEC—476*

The paradoxical movement is due to the instability of the chest wall. During inspiration, the negative pressures within the chest wall cause the flail segment to suck in. Upon exhalation, the positive intrathoracic pressures cause the flail segment to bow out. These movements are the opposite of how the the rest of the chest wall moves.

Figure 16-2

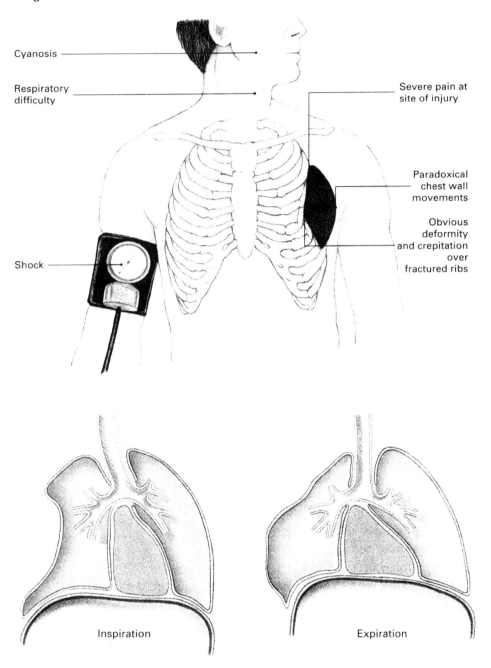

Cyanosis

Respiratory difficulty

Shock

Severe pain at site of injury

Paradoxical chest wall movements

Obvious deformity and crepitation over fractured ribs

Inspiration

Expiration

Source: PEC, Figures 16-3 and 16-4.

23. ANS—D   *PEC—476*

Flail chest can result in severe respiratory compromise. The hypoventilation results in decreased air available for gas exchange, leading to hypoxia and hypercarbia. Broken rib pieces can also cause penetrating injuries to the lungs.

24. ANS—A *PEC—491*

Prehospital management of a patient suspected of having a flail chest includes positive pressure ventilation to ensure good ventilation and stabilizing a loose flail segment.

25. ANS—B *PEC—478*

This patient who presents with absent lung sounds on one side with decreased sounds on the other, with hyperressonance, jugular venous distention, and a deviated trachea has a tension pneumothorax.

26. ANS—D *PEC—478*

Her hypotension could be the result of a combination of factors. The high intrathoracic pressures caused by the injury may decrease venous return. The tension could produce a tamponade effect on the heart, severely decreasing cardiac output. She may have blood loss from bleeding within the chest or other injuries.

Figure 16-3

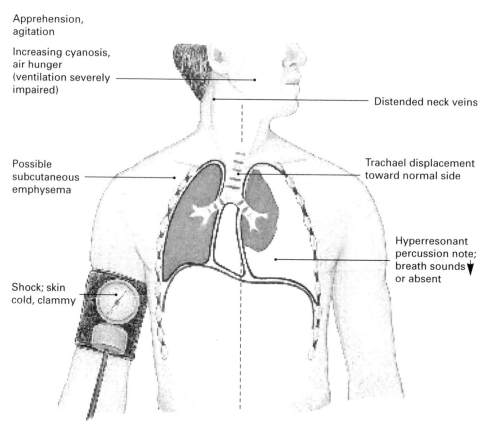

Apprehension, agitation

Increasing cyanosis, air hunger (ventilation severely impaired)

Distended neck veins

Possible subcutaneous emphysema

Trachael displacement toward normal side

Hyperresonant percussion note; breath sounds▼ or absent

Shock; skin cold, clammy

Source: PEC, Figure 16-5.

27. ANS—B *PEC—493*

Emergency management of this patient includes immediate and rapid evacuation of the air trapped in the pleural space. Needle decompression is done by placing a large bore IV catheter into the chest at the second intercostal space, midclavicular line. Then, remove the needle and attach a one-way valve device allowing air to escape, but not enter.

Figure 16-4

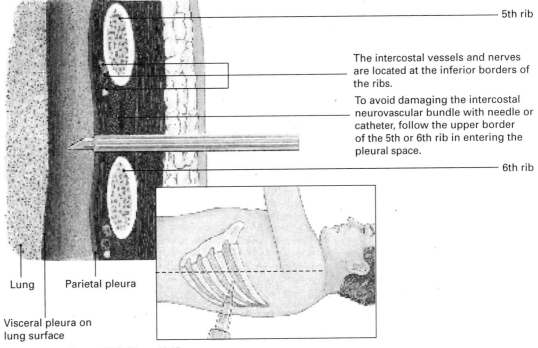

5th rib

The intercostal vessels and nerves are located at the inferior borders of the ribs.

To avoid damaging the intercostal neurovascular bundle with needle or catheter, follow the upper border of the 5th or 6th rib in entering the pleural space.

6th rib

Lung   Parietal pleura

Visceral pleura on lung surface

Source: PEC, Figure 16-15.

28. ANS—B   *PEC—478*

This patient's presentation of dyspnea, pain to the right chest, diminished breath sounds on the right side, dull to percussion on the right side, and shock indicate hemothorax. A hemothorax is caused by bleeding into the pleural space.

Figure 16-5

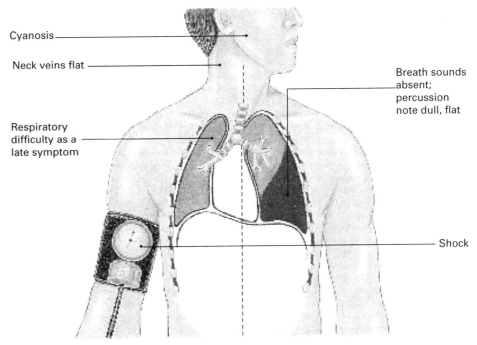

Cyanosis

Neck veins flat

Breath sounds absent; percussion note dull, flat

Respiratory difficulty as a late symptom

Shock

Source: PEC, Figure 16-6.

29. ANS—A   *PEC—489*

Emergency field management of this patient includes treating for shock by replacing blood fluid volume rapidly.

30. ANS—D   *PEC—480*

This patient's presentation of distant heart sounds, distended neck veins, and a narrow pulse pressure indicate pericardial tamponade. This is the classic "Beck's Triad."

31. ANS—B   *PEC—480*

Pericardial tamponade is the filling of the pericardial sac with fluid which in turn limits the filling of the heart.

Figure 16-6

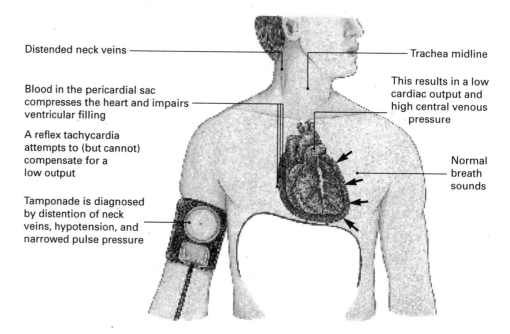

Distended neck veins

Trachea midline

This results in a low cardiac output and high central venous pressure

Blood in the pericardial sac compresses the heart and impairs ventricular filling

A reflex tachycardia attempts to (but cannot) compensate for a low output

Normal breath sounds

Tamponade is diagnosed by distention of neck veins, hypotension, and narrowed pulse pressure

Source: PEC, Figure 16-7.

32. ANS—D   *PEC—494*

Definitive emergency management of this patient includes pericardiocentesis. This procedure involves the insertion of a large bore spinal needle into the pericardial sac and aspirating the excess blood. This procedure has many complications and is seldom performed by paramedics in the field. This patient requires rapid transport.

33. ANS—C   *PEC—481*

Any patient who presents with signs and symptoms of shock and discoloration around the umbilicus, also known as Cullen's sign, should be suspected of having an intraabdominal hemorrhage.

34. ANS—C   *PEC—485*

The peritoneum can become irritated by the presence of blood. The patient with peritoneal irritation often presents with guarding because it hurts to move.

35. ANS—D   *PEC—496*

Field management of this patient includes the pneumatic anti-shock garment, IV fluid replacement, and rapid transport to a trauma center.

CHAPTER 17

Musculoskeletal Trauma

QUESTIONS

1. Which of the following is NOT part of the axial skeleton?
A. Skull
B. Pelvis
C. Vertebral column
D. Thorax

Match the following components of long bones with their definitions:

2. _____ Diaphysis   A. Intermediate transition region

3. _____ Epiphysis   B. Passages for blood vessels and nerves

4. _____ Metaphysis   C. The wide end of a long bone

5. _____ Periosteum   D. Long cylindrical shaft

6. _____ Haversian canals   E. Tough outer bone layer

7. Connective tissue that provides the articular surfaces of the skeletal system is called
A. cartilage
B. synovium
C. ligament
D. fossa

8. Connective tissue bands which hold joints together are called
A. fossa

    B. ligaments
    C. cartilage
    D. synovium

9. The oily, viscous fluid that lubricates articular surfaces is known as
    A. fossa
    B. ligaments
    C. cartilage
    D. synovium

10. The most commonly fractured bone in the human body is the
    A. scapula
    B. humerus
    C. femur
    D. clavicle

11. The proximal humerus articulates with the
    A. radius
    B. ulna
    C. glenoid fossa
    D. clavicle

12. The act of turning the palm or foot upward is called
    A. pronation
    B. abduction
    C. adduction
    D. supination

13. The metacarpal bones articulate with the
    A. radius
    B. ulna
    C. phalanges
    D. all of the above

14. The hollow surface of the pelvis into which the head of the femur fits is the
    A. glenoid fossa
    B. calcaneus
    C. acetabulum
    D. tibial plateau

15. The distal femur articulates with the
    A. pelvis
    B. tibia
    C. fibula
    D. radius

16. The medial malleolus is formed by the
    A. tibia
    B. fibula
    C. calcaneus
    D. tarsal bones

17. _____ is the only muscle over which we have control.

A. Cardiac muscle
B. Smooth muscle
C. Skeletal muscle
D. None of the above

18. The Achilles is an example of a
A. ligament
B. tendon
C. cartilage
D. long bone

19. Blunt trauma causing bleeding and discoloration underneath the skin is a
A. laceration
B. contusion
C. abrasion
D. subluxation

20. Overstretching of a muscle is called a
A. strain
B. sprain
C. subluxation
D. dislocation

21. Overstretching of a ligament is known as a/an
A. strain
B. sprain
C. abduction
D. adduction

22. A partial separation of a joint is called a/an
A. dislocation
B. subluxation
C. pronation
D. insufflation

Match the following fractures with their respective definitions:

23. _____ Hairline   **A.** Partial break on one side of bone only
24. _____ Comminuted   **B.** Bone ends compress together
25. _____ Impacted   **C.** Complete break across bone
26. _____ Greenstick   **D.** Bone ends fragmented
27. _____ Oblique   **E.** Diagonal break
28. _____ Transverse   **F.** Small crack in the bone

29. Often you may not be able to differentiate a proximal femur fracture from a/an
A. posterior hip dislocation
B. anterior hip dislocation
C. pelvic fracture
D. acetabulum fracture

30. Colle's fracture involves which bone(s)?
   A. Proximal ulna
   B. Proximal radius
   C. Distal radius
   D. Distal ulna

31. Which of the following statements is true regarding the management of musculoskeletal injuries?
   A. Always splint the joints above and below the fracture site.
   B. Always splint the bones above and below a dislocated joint.
   C. Always perform distal neurovascular tests before and after any splinting.
   D. All of the above.

32. The management of a pelvic fracture includes which of the following procedures?
   A. Pneumatic antishock garment
   B. IV fluid replacement
   C. Immobilization of the pelvic ring
   D. All of the above

33. Traction splinting is indicated in which of the following conditions?
   A. Isolated midshaft femur fracture
   B. Disease-induced proximal femur fracture
   C. Bilateral femur fractures with profound shock
   D. All of the above

34. When should you attempt to manipulate a knee dislocation?
   A. Always
   B. Never
   C. If distal pulses are absent
   D. If the patient experiences pain

35. In which of the following cases would the pneumatic antishock garment be an effective splint?
   A Pelvic fracture
   B. Bilateral femur fractures
   C. Tibia / fibula fracture with extensive bleeding
   D. All of the above

ANSWERS   **1. ANS—B**   *PEC—501*

The axial skeleton consists of the skull, the vertebral column, and the thorax. The upper and lower extremities, the shoulder girdle, and the pelvis make up the appendicular skeleton.

2. ____ Diaphysis	**D.** Long cylindrical shaft
3. ____ Epiphysis	**C.** The wide end of a long bone
4. ____ Metaphysis	**A.** Intermediate transition region
5. ____ Periosteum	**E.** Tough outer bone layer
6. ____ Haversian canals	**B.** Passages for blood vessels and nerves

7. ANS—A   *PEC—503*

A layer of connective tissue called cartilage covers the epiphyseal surface. It is a smooth, strong, flexible material that functions as the actual surface of articulation between bones. It allows for easy movements between the ends of adjacent bones, such as the femur and tibia. It also absorbs some of the impact associated with walking, running, or other jarring activities.

8. ANS—B   *PEC—504*

Ligaments are connective tissues connecting bone to bone and holding the joints together. Ligaments will stretch to allow joint movement while holding the bone ends firmly in place.

9. ANS—D   *PEC—504*

The ligaments surrounding a joint form the synovial capsule. This chamber holds a small amount of fluid to lubricate the articular surfaces. The oily viscus fluid assists joint motion by reducing friction.

10. ANS—D   *PEC—504*

The clavicle which is anterior to the scapula and not very well protected is the most commonly fractured bone in the human body.

11. ANS—C   *PEC—504*

The humerus is the single bone of the proximal upper extremity. It is secured against the glenoid fossa of the shoulder joint proximally. The humerus articulates with the radius and ulna at the elbow.

12. ANS—D   *PEC—504*

The act of turning the palm or foot upward is called supination. The opposite movement, turning the hand or foot downward is called pronation.

13. ANS—C   *PEC—504*

The metacarpal bones articulate with the phalanges of the fingers and the carpal bones.

14. ANS—C   *PEC—504*

The actual articular surface for the femur is the acetabulum. It is a hollow depression in the lateral pelvis into which the head of the femur fits.

15. ANS—B   *PEC—505*

The distal femur articulates with the tibia.

16. ANS—A   *PEC—505*

The distal tibia forms the medial malleolus or the protruberance of the ankle while the fibia forms the lateral malleolus.

17. ANS—C   *PEC—505*

Skeletal muscles are muscles over which we have conscious control. They are necessary to move the extremities and the body in general. The largest component of the muscular system, they are the muscles most commonly traumatized.

18. ANS—B   *PEC—505*

The Achilles is an example of a tendon. A tendon is a specialized connective tissue band that accomplishes the insertion and in some cases the origin of muscles. They are extremely strong and will not stretch and in many instances. They often will break an area of bone loose rather than tear.

19. ANS—B *PEC—506*

Trauma frequently causes contusion. As with all contusions, small blood vessels rupture causing dull pain, leakage of fluid into the interstitial spaces, and the classical discoloration.

20. ANS—A *PEC—507*

A strain is an overstretching of the muscle and presents as pain.

21. ANS—B *PEC—507*

The sprain is a tearing of the connective tissue of the joint capsule, specifically a ligament or ligaments. This injury causes exquisite pain at the site followed shortly by inflammation and swelling.

22. ANS—B *PEC—507*

A subluxation is an incomplete dislocation of the joint. The surfaces remain in contact while the joint is partially deformed.

23. ____	Hairline	**F.**	Small crack in the bone
24. ____	Comminuted	**D.**	Bone ends fragmented
25. ____	Impacted	**B.**	Bone ends compress together
26. ____	Greenstick	**A.**	Partial break on one side of bone only
27. ____	Oblique	**E.**	Diagonal break
28. ____	Transverse	**C.**	Complete break across bone

29. ANS—B *PEC—511*

Fracture of the femur near the hip may be difficult to differentiate from an anterior hip dislocation. While you may expect a broken leg to be slightly shorter than the unbroken one, the difference may be slight and unnoticeable if the legs are not straight and parallel.

30. ANS—C *PEC—512*

Commonly fractures will occur at the distal end of the radius breaking it just above the articular surface. This is known as a Colle's fracture and presents with the wrist turned up at an unusual angle.

31. ANS—D *PEC—516*

Always splint the joints above and below the fracture site and the bones above and below a dislocated joint. Before and after any splinting always perform distal neurovascular checks checking for circulation, sensory, and motor function.

32. ANS—D *PEC—517*

Management of a pelvic fracture includes pneumatic anti-shock garment, immobilizing the pelvic ring, and rapid IV fluid replacement.

33. ANS—A *PEC—518*

The traction splint is the best device to splint the hemodynamically stable patient with an isolated femur fracture.

34. ANS—C *PEC—518*

As a rule, immobilize knee dislocations as you find them unless you cannot palpate distal pulses. In this case, manipulate the limb until the pulse returns or the patient experiences extreme pain.

35. ANS—D   *PEC—517*

The pneumatic antishock garment is an excellent splinting device that also tamponades bleeding underneath the suit. It can be an effective device for splinting pelvic fractures, bilateral femur fractures, and any lower extremity fracture with extensive bleeding.

CHAPTER 18

Soft Tissue Trauma and Burns

QUESTIONS

1. The outermost layer of the skin consisting of dead or dying cells is the
  A. epidermis
  B. dermis
  C. subcutaneous layer
  D. sebacous layer

2. Fatty secretion that helps keep the skin pliable and waterproof is called
  A. intima
  B. cilia
  C. mucus
  D. sebum

3. The skin layer containing blood vessels and nerves is the
  A. epidermis
  B. dermis
  C. subcutaneous layer
  D. sebacous layer

4. The layer containing adipose fat and and connective tissue is the
  A. epidermis
  B. dermis
  C. subcutaneous layer
  D. sebacous layer

5. The smooth interior layer of the blood vessels is the tunica
    A. intima
    B. media
    C. adventitia
    D. lumina

6. The middle, muscular layer of the blood vessels is the tunica
    A. intima
    B. media
    C. adventitia
    D. lumina

7. The outer fibrous layer of the blood vessels is the tunica
    A. intima
    B. media
    C. adventitia
    D. lumina

8. The functions of the skin include
    A. protecting the body from environmental pathogens
    B. providing a barrier against infection
    C. perceiving temperature, pain, and pressure
    D. all of the above

9. A closed wound in which the skin is unbroken, but the tissue underneath is damaged is a/an
    A. abrasion
    B. concussion
    C. contusion
    D. amputation

10. General reddening of the skin due to dilation of the superficial capillaries is
    A. ecchymosis
    B. erythema
    C. hyphema
    D. contusion

11. A scraping away of the superficial layers of the skin is a/an
    A. erythema
    B. ecchymosis
    C. contusion
    D. abrasion

12. A collection of blood trapped within a body compartment is a/an
    A. hyphema
    B. erythema
    C. hematoma
    D. contusion

13. Black and blue discoloration of the skin due to leakage of blood into the tissues is
    A. hyphema

    B. ecchymosis

    C. erythema

    D. contusion

14. In the healthy adult, the clotting mechanism takes about

    A. 5 minutes

    B. 10 minutes

    C. 20 minutes

    D. 30 minutes

15. The extent of burn injury depends upon which of the following factors?

    A. Temperature

    B. Concentration of heat energy

    C. Length of contact time

    D. All of the above

16. Which of the following types of radiation emits the most powerful rays

    A. Alpha

    B. Beta

    C. Delta

    D. Gamma

17. The extent of radiation depends on which of the following factors?

    A. Duration of exposure

    B. Distance from the source

    C. Shielding from the source

    D. All of the above

18. Your patient who presents with dyspnea and hoarseness, following the inhalation of superheated steam is in danger of developing

    A. pulmonary embolism

    B. complete airway obstruction

    C. anaphylaxis

    D. pulmonary edema

19. Any patient who has been in an enclosed area during combustion should be suspected of having

    A. pulmonary embolism

    B. pulmonary edema

    C. carbon monoxide poisoning

    D. hyponatremia

20. A burn involving the epidermis and dermis, producing blisters and pain is classified as

    A. first degree

    B. second degree

    C. third degree

    D. fourth degree

21. An adult with burns to both arms, chest, abdomen, and entire back has a _____% BSA burn.

    A. 36

    B. 45

    C. 54
    D. 63

22. A child with burns to both legs has a ____% BSA burn.
    A. 9
    B. 14
    C. 18
    D. 28

23. Which of the following is a complication of a burn injury?
    A. Hypothermia
    B. Hypovolemia
    C. Eschar
    D. All of the above

24. The major complication of circumferential burns is the
    A. fluid loss in the burn area
    B. loss of barrier against infection
    C. tourniquet effect cutting off distal circulation
    D. anaerobic metabolism proximal to the burn site

25. An example of a burn injury that should be evaluated in a burn center is
    A. second degree burn to >15% of BSA
    B. third degree burn to >5% of BSA
    C. high voltage electrical injury
    D. all of the above

26. The proper care for an amputated part includes placing the part
    A. directly on ice
    B. in warm saline
    C. in a sealed dry bag, then into cold water
    D. directly into cold water

27. What perecntage of partial thickness burns can be safely cooled with water?
    A. 10%
    B. 20%
    C. 25%
    D. 50%

28. Partial thickness burns over 30% or full thickness burns over 5% of BSA should be managed by
    A. rapid cooling with water
    B. water and fanning
    C. applying ice to the burned area
    D. dry, sterile dresings

29. Standard management of chemical burns includes
    A. rinsing the area with ice water
    B. using a neutralizing agent
    C. leaving any corrosive materials on the skin
    D. vigorous irrigation with cool water

30. Which of the following substances can you safely irrigate?
A. Sodium
B. Phenol
C. Lye
D. Dry lime

ANSWERS

1. ANS—A   *PEC—523*

The outermost layer of skin is the epidermis. It is composed of dead or dying cells that are pushed outward by new cells growing underneath. As these cells reach the surface, they wear away with everyday activity.

2. ANS—D   *PEC—523*

Sebum is the fatty secretion from the sebaceous gland. This oil lubricates the the epidermis and helps make it both pliable and watertight.

3. ANS—B   *PEC—524*

The dermis is the layer of tissue that contains blood vessels, nerves, sweat glands, sebaceous glands, and hair follicles.

4. ANS—C   *PEC—524*

The subcutaneous layer is comprised of fat and connective tissue and serves to insulate the body.

5. ANS—A   *PEC—524*

The tunica intima is the smooth, thin lining of blood vessels. It allows for free flow of blood and promotes the exchange of nutrients and waste products between the tissues and the bloodstream.

6. ANS—B   *PEC—525*

The tunica media is the muscular part of the tube. It regulates the inner diameter of the blood vessel by either dilating or constricting to meet the body's demands. These involuntary muscles are under the control of the autonomic nervous system.

7. ANS—C   *PEC—525*

The tunica adventitia is the outer fibrous layer of the blood vessels. This layer consists of connective tissue and provides protection.

8. ANS—D   *PEC—525*

The functions of the skin are many. It protects the human body from many dangers found in the environment; functions as an organ of sensation, perceiving temperature and pain; contains vital fluids; aids in temperature regulation through secretion of sweat and shunting of blood; and provides a barrier against infection and insulation from trauma.

9. ANS—C   *PEC—525*

A contusion is a closed wound in which the skin is unbroken although damage has occurred to the immediate tissue beneath. It is usually caused by blunt, non-penetrating injuries that crush and damage small blood vessels.

10. ANS—B   *PEC—526*

An erythema is general reddening of the skin due to dilation of the superficial capillaries. This situation is often caused by a contusion.

11. ANS—D *PEC—526*

An abrasion is the scraping away of the superficial layers of the skin often by an open soft tissue injury. An abrasion removes the layers of the epidermis and upper reaches of the dermis. Bleeding is usually limited because the injury involves only superficial capillaries.

12. ANS—C *PEC—526*

A hematoma is a collection of blood beneath the skin or trapped within a body compartment. Hematomas can contribute significantly to hypovolemia. For example, the thigh can contain over a liter of fluid before swelling becomes apparent.

13. ANS—B *PEC—526*

Ecchymosis is the black and blue discoloration of the skin caused by leakage of blood into the tissues. It is a delayed sign in wound progression.

14. ANS—B *PEC—528*

The clotting mechanism takes about 10 minutes in the normal, healthy adult. It is more rapid if the injury involves a small vessel. It is less rapid if the vessel is a large artery or vein.

15. ANS—D *PEC—529*

The extent of burn injury depends upon the amount of heat energy transfered to the patient's body. When assessing the severity of a burn injury focus on three important factors: the temperature, the concentration of heat energy, and the length of contact time.

16. ANS—D *PEC—531*

Gamma radiation, also known as x-rays, is the most powerful ionizing radiation. It has the ability to travel through the entire body or ionize any atom within. It is the most dangerous and most feared type of radiation because it is difficult to protect against.

17. ANS—D *PEC—531*

The extent of a radiation injury depends upon three important factors: the duration of the exposure, the distance from the source, and the shielding from the source.

18. ANS—B *PEC—532*

A patient who inhales superheated steam and presents with shortness of breath, difficulty breathing, and hoarseness is in danger of developing a complete airway obstruction. Superheated steam contains enough energy to severely burn the upper airway. If damaged, this tissue will swell rapidly and seriously reduce the size of the airway lumen. The patient who presents with minor hoarseness may develop a complete airway obstruction later on.

19. ANS—C *PEC—533*

Any patient who has been in an enclosed area during combustion should be suspected of having carbon monoxide poisoning. Carbon monoxide is a by-product of incomplete combustion. Poisoning occurs because the hemoglobin of the blood has a much greater infinity for carbon monoxide than it does for oxygen. If your patient inhales carbon monoxide, it will displace oxygen with resulting hypoxemia.

20. ANS—B   *PEC—533*

A second degree burn involves the epidermis and the dermis. It produces blisters and is extremely painful.

Characteristics of Various Depths of Burns

	First Degree	Second Degree	Third Degree
Cause	Sun or minor flash	Hot liquids, flashes, or flame	Chemicals, electricity, flame, hot metals
Skin color	Red	Mottled red	Pearly white and/or charred, translucent, and parchment-like
Skin	Dry with no surface blister	Blisters with weeping	Dry with thrombosed blood vessels
Sensation	Painful	Painful	Anesthetic
Healing	3–6 days	2–4 weeks, depending on depth	Requires skin grafting

21. ANS—C   *PEC—535*

The rule of nines states that in the adult patient the arms are worth 9, the chest and abdomen 18, and the entire back 18. This patient, therefore, has a 54% BSA burn.

Figure 18-1

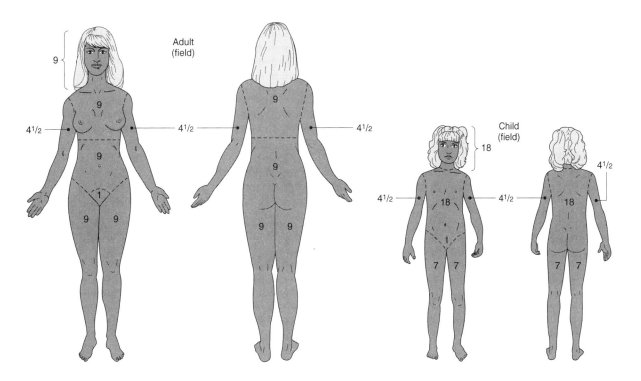

Source: PEC, Figure 18-12.

22. ANS—D *PEC—535*

In the child the rule of nines differs slightly. The head being larger in proportion to the rest of the body is worth 18%. The legs, therefore, are 14% each. So a child with burns to both legs has a 28% BSA burn.

23. ANS—D *PEC—536*

Some complications of burns include hypothermia (loss of body heat through the burn area), hypovolemia (plasma loss through the burn area), and eschar (destroyed skin cells).

24. ANS—C *PEC—537*

A circumferential burn encircles the complete exterior of an extremity. In these types of burns the constriction may be severe enough to include all blood flow into the distal extremity. In the case of a thoracic burn it may drastically reduce chest expansion reducing respiratory title volume.

25. ANS—D *PEC—542*

Injuries that benefit from Burn Center Care are listed in the following table:

Injuries that Benefit from Burn Center Care
A. Second-degree burn greater than 15 percent of body surface area (BSA)   **B.** Third-degree burn greater than 5 percent BSA   **C.** Significant face, feet, hands, perineal burns   **D.** High-voltabe electrical injury   **E.** Inhalation injury   **F.** Chemical burns causing progressive tissue destruction   **G.** Associated significant injuries
Source: American Burn Association

26. ANS—C *PEC—546*

Current recommendations for managing amputated body parts includes dry cooling and rapid transport. Place the amputated part in a plastic bag and keep it cool by cold water immersion. The water in which the bag and the body part sits may have ice cubes in it, but avoid direct contact between the ice and the injured part.

27. ANS—A *PEC—548*

Use local cooling to treat minor soft tissue burns that involve only a small portion of the body surface area at partial thickness. Care for only those burns that involve less than 10% of the body surface area in this way.

28. ANS—D *PEC—548*

Use dry sterile dressings to treat partial thickness burns over 30% of the body or full thickness burns over 5% of the body surface area. This will reduce air movement past the sensitive first and second degree burns and provide padding against minor bumping. In the third degree burn they provide a barrier to possible contamination.

29. ANS—A *PEC—548*

Prehospital management of most chemical burns includes rinsing the area with large volumes of cool water. The water not only rinses away the offending material, but also dilutes any water soluble agents. The cooling affect of the water also reduces the heat and the rate of chemical reaction.

30. ANS—C   *PEC—549*

Some substances either do not dissolve in water or may react violently with it. Phenol, dry lime, and sodium are three of those substances. All others should be irrigated with copious amounts of water.

CHAPTER 19

Shock Trauma Resuscitation

QUESTIONS

SCENARIO Your patient was the driver in a one-car high speed auto accident involving frontal impact with a telephone pole. He is a 19-year-old male who presents unconscious and partially trapped in the severely deformed vehicle. According to witnesses, he was driving at a high rate of speed. Upon initial examination, you immediately hear gurgling respirations. Vital signs are: weak carotid pulse rate of 120, BP—70/40, respiratory rate is 36 and shallow, skin cool, pale, and clammy, capillary refill time is :04 seconds. Pulse oximetry reads 70%. Upon physical exam, you discover a bruise to the front chest wall with loose flail segment and some abdominal guarding. Lung sounds are diminished on the right side with some hyperressonance in that area.

1. Which of the following conditions indicates the need to rapidly transport your patient to a trauma center?
A. Severe deformity to his vehicle
B. His respiratory rate
C. His systolic blood pressure
D. All of the above

2. Your initial management of this patient should be to
A. perform immediate nasotracheal intubation

    B. start two large bore IVs
    C. manually stabilize his head and neck
    D. place an oxygen mask on him

3. The gurgling noise that accompanies his breathing calls for immediate
    A. suctioning
    B. intubation
    C. head-tilt/chin lift procedure
    D. chest decompression

4. You are concerned about the right-sided flail segment because
    A. it indicates lung tissue damage beneath the injury
    B. it severely inhibits ventilation and oxygenation
    C. it is usually accompanied by pericardial tamponade
    D. underlying damage to the heart is expected

5. His respiratory situation indicates the need for immediate
    A. chest decompression
    B. Trendelenberg positioning
    C. intubation
    D. positive pressure ventilation

6. Your patient's pulse and blood pressure indicate which stage of shock?
    A. Compensated
    B. Irreversible
    C. Decompensated
    D. None of the above

7. The most likely cause of your patient's shock is
    A. loss of alveoli function
    B. internal blood loss
    C. massive vasodilation
    D. acute myocardial infarction

8. Peripheral vascular resistance is regulated in which blood vessels?
    A. veins
    B. venules
    C. arteries
    D. arterioles

9. Which of the following statements is TRUE regarding this patient?
    A. Anaerobic metabolism is occurring
    B. Resuscitation is still possible
    C. Irreversible shock will ensue if left untreated
    D. All of the above

10. This patient responds to pain stimuli by moaning. He earns a _____ on the AVPU scale.
    A. A
    B. V
    C. P
    D. U

11. If used, the pneumatic antishock garment should have the following beneficial effects:
   A. autotransfusion of over 1000 ml of blood to the vital organs
   B. decrease peripheral resistance to enhance circulation
   C. tamponade internal abdominal hemorrhage
   D. stop the anaerobic metabolism from progressing

12. Prehospital management fluid resuscitation of this patient should include
   A. Lactated Ringer's
   B. 0.45% sodium chloride
   C. 5% dextrose and water
   D. any of the above

13. Which of the following IV equipment would best help this patient?
   A. 20 gauge, 2 inch catheter, 60 drop/ml tubing
   B. 14 gauge, 1 inch catheter, 10 drop/ml tubing
   C. 16 gauge, 3 inch catheter, 60 drop/ml tubing
   D. 22 gauge, 1/2 inch catheter, 10 drop/ml tubing

14. By using a 12 gauge catheter instead of a 24 gauge catheter, you will flow fluid
   A. twice as fast
   B. twice as slow
   C. 16 times as fast
   D. 8 times slower

15. Infusing three liters of fluid into this patient will raise his intravascular blood volume by
   A. 3 liters
   B. 6 liters
   C. 2 liters
   D. 1 liter

16. Fluid resuscitation in the field should be limited to
   A. 1 liter
   B. 2 liters
   C. 3 liters
   D. none of the above

17. The Seldinger technique is used to
   A. infuse fluids under pressure
   B. attach the IV bag directly to the blood tubing
   C. place large bore catheters peripherally
   D. deflate the PASG

18. During a hot load, you should always
   A. approach the helicopter from the rear
   B. stay clear of the tail rotor
   C. direct lights directly at the pilot
   D. use flares instead of flashlights

19. The appropriate helicopter landing zone for a large aircraft is
   A. 60 × 60
   B. 75 × 75
   C. 120 × 120
   D. 200 × 200

20. Which of the following criteria is important in establishing a landing zone?
   A. Level ground
   B. Clear of debris
   C. Free of wires and trees
   D. All of the above

ANSWERS

1. ANS—D   *PEC—563*

This patient has three criteria that indicate rapid transport to a trauma center: a severe deformity to his vehicle, a respiratory rate of 36, and a systolic blood pressure of 70.

2. ANS—C   *PEC—560*

Always stabilize a cervical spine if the mechanism of injury strongly suggests an injury in this area. Assign one of your crew to stabilize the head manually while you continue your primary assessment. Release manual stabilization only after you secure the head to a long spine board.

3. ANS—A   *PEC—560*

Always ensure a patent airway immediately. Examine it for fluids, obstruction, or signs of trauma and apply suction as necessary. A noisy airway is an obstructive airway.

4. ANS—B   *PEC—560*

Always be concerned about a flail segment because it may severly inhibit ventilation and oxygenation. Your patient may become hypoxic and hypercarbic.

5. ANS—D   *PEC—560*

This patient's respiratory situation indicates the need for positive pressure ventilation with a bag-valve mask and supplemental oxygen.

6. ANS—C   *PEC—559*

Your patient's blood pressure and pulse indicate that he is in decompensated shock. It's during this stage that the body's normal defense mechanisms are failing.

7. ANS—B   *PEC—561*

The most probable cause of this patient's shock is internal blood loss, probably in the abdomen.

8. ANS—D   *PEC—556*

Peripheral vascular resistence is regulated in the arterioles. Arterioles have the ability to affect blood pressure and direct blood flow from the heart to various organs. They can open and close with a valve-like function and can vary their inner diameter by as much as a factor of five.

9. ANS—D   *PEC—558*

In decompensated shock anaerobic metabolism occurs. Anaerobic metabolism occurs when there is insufficient oxygen for the cell to function. As a result of this inefficient process, acids accumulate. Resuscitation at this point is still possible, but irreversible shock will ensue if this patient is left untreated.

10. ANS—C   *PEC—562*

Since this patient only responds to pain stimuli, he earns a P on the AVPU scale.

11. ANS—C   *PEC—565*

By inflating the pneumatic antishock garment, you will tamponade the internal abdominal hemorrhage.

12. ANS—A   *PEC—567*

Prehospital fluid resuscitation is accomplished using normal saline or Lactated Ringer's. These isotonic solutions are most ideal for fluid resuscitation because they tend to remain in the intravascular space for a period of time.

13. ANS—B   *PEC—566*

In order to maximize fluid flow, use an IV catheter with the largest gauge and shortest length, and 10 drop per milliliter IV tubing.

14. ANS—C   *PEC—566*

Fluid flow is a factor of catheter diameter to a power of four, as described in Poiseulle's law. By doubling the internal diameter of a catheter, the fluid will flow 16 times faster.

15. ANS—D   *PEC—567*

There are limits to the effectiveness to the crystalloided infusions. Infusing three liters of crystalloid will expand the intravascular blood volume by only one liter. This is because much of the fluid leaks from the capillaries into the interstitial and intracellular spaces.

16. ANS—C   *PEC—567*

Crystalloid infusion, such as lactated Ringer's and normal saline, is not a complete replacement for blood. It does not contain either the hemoglobin needed to carry oxygen to the body cells or the clotting factors. Infusing more than three liters of crystalloid may severly dilute the blood so it does not carry enough hemoglobin and will not clot effectively.

17. ANS—C   *PEC—566*

Placement of a large bore catheter can be difficult in a normotensive patient, much less one in shock. A procedure that facilitates IV insertion is the Seldinger technique. It involves normal peripheral venipuncture using a moderately sized over-the-needle catheter. Once the catheter is in place the needle is withdrawn and a guide wire is passed through it. The catheter is then withdrawn and a dilater and a number 8 or 9 French catheter are threaded along the wire guide into the vein. The wire and dilater are removed leaving the large catheter in place. The technique is simple, quite effective, and allows for the passage of a large catheter into a relatively small peripheral vein.

18. ANS—B   *PEC—569*

Hot loading refers to loading a patient into a helicopter while the rotors continue to turn. If you are asked to help load the patient, stay close to the flight crew, and avoid the area of the tail rotor. The tail rotor spins at speeds in excess of 2000 rpm and is almost invisible.

19. ANS—C   *PEC—568*

A landing zone should be a minimum of 60×60 feet for small helicopters, 75×75 feet for medium ones, and a 120×120 feet for large ones.

20. ANS—D   *PEC—568*

The landing zone should be as level as possible and clear of slush, debris, and snow. It should also be free of wires, trees, and other obstructions that may impede landing or interfere with patient loading.

DIVISION 4—MEDICAL

CHAPTER 20

Respiratory Emergencies

QUESTIONS

1. The term that means "difficulty in breathing" is
   A. orthopnea
   B. apnea
   C. hypopnea
   D. dyspnea

2. A patient who presents with orthopnea
   A. has difficulty in breathing sitting straight up
   B. has difficulty in breathing when lying flat
   C. uses only the diaphragm
   D. depends on hypoxic drive to breathe

3. Coughing up blood from the respiratory tree is called
   A. hematemesis
   B. hematoma
   C. hymoptysis
   D. hymenoptera

4. Pulsus paradoxus occurs when
   A. the pulse increases during inspiration
   B. the systolic BP decreases 10 torr while breathing
   C. the pulse rises and blood pressure drops when the patient sits up
   D. none of the above

5. Vibratory tremors felt through the chest by palpation is called
   A. percussive tremors
   B. tactile fremitus
   C. bronchophony
   D. pectoriloquy

6. Your patient who presents with shortness of breath, chest pain, fever, chills, general malaise, with productive yellow sputum streaked with blood, rales and wheezes in the right lower lobe probably has
   A. congestive heart failure
   B. emphysema
   C. an acute asthma attack
   D. pneumonia

7. The problem described in question 6 is a respiratiory infection caused by
   A. a virus
   B. a bacteria
   C. a fungus
   D. all of the above

8. Which of the following could be the result of inhalating superheated steam?
   A. Laryngospasm and upper airway edema
   B. Bronchospasm and lower airway edema
   C. Pulmonary edema
   D. All of the above

9. Your first concern in dealing with any patient with a suspected toxic inhalation injury is
   A. managing the airway
   B. administering 100% oxygen
   C. your own personal safety
   D. removing the patient from the course

SCENARIO Your patient is a firefighter who took off his self-contained breathing apparatus (SCBA) while performing overhaul procedures in a house fire. He presents with a headache, irritability, loss of coordination, and confusion.

10. This patient is probably suffering from
   A. acute myocardial infarction
   B. carbon monoxide poisoning
   C. transient ischemic attack
   D. stroke

11. The pathophysiology of this problem includes
   A. CO binding on hemoglobin
   B. cellular hypoxia
   C. metabolic acidosis
   D. all of the above

12. Management of this situation includes
   A. Airway management
   B. 100% oxygenation
   C. transportation to a hyperbaric chamber
   D. all of the above

SCENARIO Your patient is a 45-year-old man who complains of sudden onset of upper right-sided stabbing chest pain and shortness of breath. He has no other medical history except for being hospitalized with pneumonia two weeks ago and sent home to recuperate. Earlier this week he had experienced some lower calf pain. He presents in moderate distress with the following vital signs: pulse 100, BP—140/80, respirations 28, skin warm and dry, and some expiratory wheezing in the area of chest pain.

13. Your prehospital diagnosis is
   A. acute asthma attack
   B. acute myocardial infarction
   C. acute pulmonary embolism
   D. spontaneous pneumothorax

14. This problem is chacterized by
   A. an allergic reaction
   B. coronary artery ischemia
   C. a moving blood clot
   D. a ruptured lung

15. A predisposing factor of this condition includes
   A. prolonged immobilization
   B. atherosclerosis
   C. congenital defect
   D. hyperreactive airways

SCENARIO Your patient is a 79-year-old female who presents in moderate respiratory distress. She sits upright and can only answer your questions with short phrases. She claims of having a recent cold and this worsening shortness of breath and cough. She denies any chest pain. She has a long history of breathing problems She claims to get this every year at this time and it lasts about two months. She also admits to smoking 2 packs of cigarettes each day for the past 50 years. Her vital signs are: pulse 100 and regular, BP—150/80, respiratory rate 36 and labored, skin cyanotic. You auscultate diffuse expiratory wheezes. She has a very productive cough with her sputum being a yellowish-brown and sticky. She has pitting pedal edema and ascites.

16. Your prehospital diagnosis should be
   A. acute asthma
   B. emphysema
   C. chronic bronchitis
   D. acute pulmonary embolism

17. The cause of this disease is
  A. allergies
  B. venous stasis
  C. years of toxic inhalation
  D. none of the above

18. The pathophysiology of this disease involves
  A. destruction of alveolar walls
  B. increased mucous production
  C. traveling blood clot
  D. hyperreactive airways

19. This patient's smoking history is described as
  A. 50 pack/years
  B. 2 pack/years
  C. 100 pack/years
  D. none of the above

20. Her sputum indicates
  A. respiratory infection
  B. pulmonary edema
  C. hematemesis
  D. hymoptysis

21. Her pedal edema is probably caused by
  A. left heart failure
  B. acute pulmonary edema
  C. peripheral vasoconstriction
  D. cor pulmonale

22. Her cyanosis is caused by
  A. hypocarbia
  B. hypoxia
  C. pulmonary hypertension
  D. increased residual volume

23. The base station physician orders you to administer albuterol via nebulizer in an attempt to
  A. decrease pulmonary edema
  B. stop the allergic reaction
  C. dilate the airways
  D. increase cardiac contractions

SCENARIO Your patient is a 24 year old male who presents in severe respiratory distress. His wife states that he has had increasing difficulty in breathing all morning but now is much worse. He has a history of asthma and takes the following oral medications: Theodur® (theophylline) and prednisone; and the following metered dose inhalers: Ventolin® (albuterol), and Beclovent® (beclomethasone). Upon examination you find an otherwise healthy person who speaks in words only. His vital signs are: pulse—120 and strong, BP—140/80, respirations 40 and very labored, skin pale. You auscultate inspiratory and expiratory wheezes and rhonchi bilaterally. He is hyperressonant to percussion.

24. Asthma is a disease characterized by
   A. airway edema
   B. bronchospasm
   C. hypermucous secretion
   D. all of the above

25. The above reactions are caused by the
   A. sympathetic nervous system response
   B. release of norepinephrine
   C. release of histamine
   D. blockage of parasympathetic action

26. Prednisone and beclomethasone are drugs that
   A. dilate the bronchioles directly
   B. decrease inflammation
   C. stimulate the respiratory center
   D. block the allergic response

27. Albuterol and theophylline are prescribed to
   A. dilate the bronchioles directly
   B. decrease inflammation
   C. inhibit the respiratory center
   D. block the allergic response

28. The hyperresonance is due to
   A. collapsed alveoli
   B. associated pneumothorax
   C. air trapping in the alveoli
   D. decreased duration of the expiratory phase

29. The Wright's Meter measures
   A. peak expiratory flow
   B. residual volume
   C. oxygen saturation
   D. total lung capacity

30. Common side effects from administering albuterol and aminophylline to your patient could include
   A. increased heart rates
   B. tremors
   C. nausea and vomiting
   D. all of the above

SCENARIO Your patient is a 59-year-old male who presents sitting at the kitchen table in moderate respiratory distress. His elbows are on the table in a tripod position and he appears to be really working at breathing. Although this problem came on gradually today, his family states that he has had lung disease for a long time. He is a lifetime smoker and is on home oxygen at 2 liters/per/minute via nasal cannula. He takes Atrovent® (ipratroprium bromide) inhaler, Theolair® (theophylline), and Proventil® (albuterol) inhaler. He appears very thin and barrel chested with a pink complexion. You immediately notice the pronounced accessory muscles in his neck and chest along with retractions. He labors to breathe, pursing his lips during exhalation. His vital signs are: pulse 90, BP—140/80, respiratory rate—40, skin warm and pink, diffuse expiratory wheezes, O_2 saturation 90%.

31. Your prehospital diagnosis is
   A. asthma
   B. congestive heart failure
   C. chronic bronchitis
   D. emphysema

32. This disease is characterized by
   A. alveolar wall destruction
   B. hypermucous secretion
   C. decreased left ventricular function
   D. allergic reaction

33. His pink complexion is caused by
   A. decreased carbon dioxide levels
   B. increased oxygen levels
   C. increased red blood cell production
   D. decreased tidal volume

34. Atrovent® is a drug in which class?
   A. Sympathomimetic
   B. Corticosteroid
   C. Anticholinergic
   D. Xanthine bronchodilator

35. Immediate management of this patient includes
   A. leaving the oxygen at 2 lpm via nasal cannula
   B. bronchodilation with albuterol
   C. IV fluid replacement with normal saline
   D. all of the above

DRUG DOSE REVIEW

Drug	Adult	Pediatric
Epinephrine 1:1000		
Albuterol		
Isoetharine		
Metaproterenol		
Terbutaline		
Methylprednisolone		

ANSWERS   **1. ANS—D**   *PEC—575*

The term dyspnea means shortness of breath. It describes the patient's subjective sensation of not being able to breath.

2. ANS—B   *PEC—575*

Orthopnea is the patient's sensation of difficulty breathing while lying flat. It is a common complaint in patients with congestive heart failure.

3. ANS—C   *PEC—575*

Hemoptysis is the coughing up of blood from the respiratory tree. Hymoptysis can be caused by tumors, pulmonary emboli, and many forms of blunt or penetrating chest trauma.

4. ANS—B   *PEC—577*

Pulsus paradoxus occurs when there is a drop in the systolic blood pressure of 10 torr or more with each respiratory cycle. It is associated with chronic obstructive pulmonary disease and cardiac tamponade. As a rule, in the field, you should not take the time to look for pulsus paradoxus.

5. ANS—B   *PEC—578*

In some patients it may be appropriate to assess for tactile fremitus. This is a vibration felt in the chest during speaking. When evaluating tactile fremitus, compare one side of the chest with the other. This sign is common in pneumonia where the sound vibrations travel further through areas of lung consolidation.

6. ANS—D   *PEC—595*

A patient who presents with shortness of breath, chest pain, fever, chills, general malaise, a productive yellow sputum streaked with blood, and rales and wheezing in the right lower lobe probably has pneumonia. Pneumonia is an infection of the lungs and a common medical problem.

7. ANS—D   *PEC—595*

Pneumonia is a common respiratory disease caused when an infectious agent invades the lungs. Pneumonia's can be bacterial, viral, or fungal. It may involve part or all of the lung.

8. ANS—D   *PEC—595*

Inhalation of superheated steam can result in upper airway obstruction due to edema and laryngospasm; lower airway edema and bronchospasm; and in severe cases, disruption of the alveolar capillary membrane resulting in life-threatening pulmonary edema.

9. ANS—C   *PEC—596*

The paramedic's first concern in any toxic inhalation situation is his own personal safety.

10. ANS—B   *PEC—596*

A particular hazard for firefighters and rescue personnel is carbon monoxide poisoning. Particularly during overhaul operations when some smoldering still occurs. A smoldering fire yields much carbon monoxide.

11. ANS—D *PEC—596*

Carbon monoxide is an odorless, tasteless, and colorless gas produced from the incomplete burning of fossil fuels. Carbon monoxide easily binds to the hemoglobin molecule. Once bound, receptor sites on the hemoglobin can no longer transport oxygen to the peripheral tissues. The result is hypoxia at the cellular level and ultimately metabolic acidosis.

12. ANS—D *PEC—596*

Management of any patient suspected of having carbon monoxide poisoning includes ensuring a patent airway, providing 100% oxygen, and rapid transportation to a hyperbaric chamber. Hyperbaric oxygen increases the PaO^2 and promotes oxygen uptake on hemoglobin molecules not yet bound by carbon monoxide.

13. ANS—C *PEC—597*

This patient who complains of sudden onset of upper right-sided stabbing chest pain and shortness of breath following hospitalization and being bed-ridden for a couple of weeks and complaining of lower leg pain, probably has suffered an acute pulmonary embolism.

14. ANS—C *PEC—597*

Pulmonary embolism is a blood clot or some other particle that lodges in a pulmonary artery. The condition is potentially life-threatening because it can significantly decrease pulmonary blood flow thus leading to hypoxemia. The problem occurs when a blood clot travels up the venous circulatory system and lodges in a pulmonary artery.

15. ANS—A *PEC—597*

Factors predisposing a patient to blood clots include prolonged immobilization, thrombophlebitis, the use of certain medications, and atrial fibrillation.

16. ANS—C *PEC—585*

Your patient presents with the classic signs and symptoms of chronic bronchitis.

17. ANS—C *PEC—585*

Following prolonged exposure to cigarette smoke the number of mucous secreting cells in the respiratory tree increases producing a large quantity of sputum.

18. ANS—B *PEC—585*

The physiology of chronic bronchitis involves increased mucuous production. This increased mucous becomes a place for bacteria to grow making the patient susceptible to frequent respiratory tract infections.

19. ANS—C *PEC—584*

Every patient suspected of having lung disease should be questioned about cigarette and tobacco use. This is generally reported in pack/years. Multiply the number of cigarette packs smoked per day by the number of years smoked. This patient smoked two packs per day for 50 years making her a 100 pack year smoker (member of the Century Club).

20. ANS—A *PEC—586*

Producing yellow sputum indicates a lower respiratory infection typical of patients with exacerbations of chronic bronchitis.

21. ANS—D *PEC—583*

Patients with chronic obstructive pulmonary disease maintain chronic high levels of carbon dioxide. Carbon dioxide is a potent, pulmonary vasoconstrictor resulting in pulmonary hypertension. This condition may lead to right heart failure or cor pulmonale.

22. ANS—B *PEC—586*

Patients with chronic bronchitis tend to be overweight and cyanotic. Because of this they are referred to as "blue bloaters." This is due to the chronic hypoxia.

23. ANS—C *PEC—586*

Common first-line treatment in chronic bronchitis is to administer a sympathomimetic bronchodilator via nebulizer in an attempt to dilate the lower airways. These inhaled beta agonists include albuterol, metaproterenol, and isoetharine.

24. ANS—D *PEC—586*

Asthma is a disease characterized by lower airway edema, bronchospasm, and hypermucous secretion. This is the classic pathophysiological triad of asthma.

25. ANS—C *PEC—587*

The first phase of asthma is characterized by the release of chemical mediators such as histamine. These mediators cause contraction of the bronchial smooth muscle and leakage of fluid from the capillaries. This results in both bronchoconstriction and bronchial edema.

26. ANS—B *PEC—587*

Prednisone and beclomethasone are drugs that decease inflammation. These belong to a class known as corticosteroids.

27. ANS—A *PEC—587*

Albuterol (beta agonist) and theophylline (xanthine) are prescribed to directly dilate the bronchioles.

28. ANS—C *PEC—588*

The asthma patient may exhibit hyperresonance upon percussion. This hyperresonance is due to the collapse of the bronchioles upon exhalation trapping air in the distal airways and alveoli.

29. ANS—A *PEC—588*

The Wright's Meter measures the peak expiratory flow rate. This flow rate that occurs during a maximum exhalation and is a reliable indicator of air flow. It's used to measure asthma severity and to monitor the patient's response to therapy.

30. ANS—D *PEC—589*

Common side affects of administering bronchodilators such as albuterol and theophylline to your patient include increased heart rates, tremors, nausea, and vomiting.

31. ANS—D   PEC—583

Prehospital diagnosis of this patient should be emphysema.

32. ANS—A   PEC—584

Emphysema results from distruction of the aveolar walls distal to the terminal bronchioles. This disease is caused by exposure to noxious substances such as cigarette smoke and results in the gradual destruction of the walls of the aveoli decreasing the aveolar membrane surface area and lessening the area available for gas exchange.

33. ANS—C   PEC—585

Patients with emphysema tend to be pink in color due to polycythemia and are referred to as "pink puffers." The polycythemia occurs as an excess of red blood cells is produced.

34. ANS—C   PEC—587

Atrovent is a drug in the anticholinergic class. This class of drugs blocks the effects of acetylcholine. Acetylcholine causes bronchoconstriction. Blocking this action allows for relaxation of the smooth muscle in the airways.

35. ANS—B   PEC—584

Immediate management of this patient includes administering 100% oxygen via a non-rebreather mask and attempting to dilate the lower airways with albuterol.

DRUG DOSE REVIEW

Drug	Adult	Pediatric
Epinephrine 1:1000	0.3—0.5 mg SC	0.01 mg / kg SC
Albuterol	0.5 mg nebulized	0.15 mg / kg nebulized
Isoetharine	0.5 ml nebulized	0.5 ml nebulized
Metaproterenol	0.2—0.3 ml nebulized	0.05—0.3 ml nebulized
Terbutaline	0.25 mg SC	0.01 mg / kg SC
Methylprednisolone	125—250 mg IV	30 mcg / kg

CHAPTER 21

Cardiovascular Emergencies

QUESTIONS

1. The great vessels enter the heart through its
   A. base
   B. apex
   C. midline
   D. ventricles

2. The innermost layer of the heart which lines the chambers is the
   A. myocardium
   B. endocardium
   C. epicardium
   D. pericardium

3. The muscular layer of the heart is the
   A. myocardium
   B. endocardium
   C. epicardium
   D. pericardium

4. The visceral pericardium is contiguous with the
   A. myocardium
   B. endocardium
   C. epicardium
   D. pleura

5. The protective sac surrounding the heart is the

A. myocardium
B. endocardium
C. epicardium
D. pericardium

6. The inferior chambers are the
A. atria
B. auricles
C. ventricles
D. vesicles

7. The only arteries that carry oxygen-poor blood are the
A. coronary arteries
B. carotid arteries
C. mesenteric arteries
D. pulmonary arteries

8. The only veins that carry oxygen-rich blood are the
A. vena cava
B. pulmonary veins
C. coronary veins
D. jugular veins

9. The greatest muscle mass is found in the
A. right atrium
B. right ventricle
C. left atrium
D. left ventricle

10. Which valves are open during systole?
A. Mitral and tricuspid valves
B. Aortic and pulmonic valves
C. AV valves
D. None of the above

11. Which valves are open during diastole?
A. Mitral and tricuspid valves
B. Aortic and pulmonic valves
C. Semi-lunar valves
D. None of the above

12. The heart muscle is perfused by the
A. coronary arteries
B. cerebral arteries
C. inferior vena cava
D. subclavian arteries

13. The development of collateral circulation is possible by the presence of
A. the coronary sinus
B. the aorta
C. anastamoses
D. automaticity

14. Blood from the coronary veins empty into the

A. right atrium
B. left atrium
C. right ventricle
D. left ventricle

15. The innermost lining of the peripheral blood vessels is the
A. tunica intima
B. tunica media
C. tunica adventitia
D. none of the above

16. The muscular layer of the peripheral blood vessels is the
A. tunica intima
B. tunica media
C. tunica adventitia
D. none of the above

17. Poiseuille's Law states that blood flow through a vessel is most dependent upon the
A. pump force
B. fluid viscosity
C. vessel length
D. vessel diameter

18. Gas exchange and cellular respiration occurs at what level of the circulation system?
A. Arterioles
B. Venules
C. Arteries
D. Capillaries

19. Which of the following does **NOT** occur during diastole?
A. Ventricular filling
B. Coronary artery perfusion
C. AV valves closed
D. Atrial contraction

20. The amount of blood ejected by the heart in one contraction is called
A. preload
B. cardiac output
C. blood pressure
D. stroke volume

21. Which of the following does **NOT** directly affect stroke volume?
A. Preload
B. Afterload
C. Heart rate
D. Contractile force

22. Up to a point, the greater the preload, the greater the
A. contractile force
B. heart rate
C. afterload

    D. blood pressure

23. The resistance against which the heart must pump is called
    A. preload
    B. afterload
    C. Starling's affect
    D. end-diastolic volume

24. Another name for preload is
    A. afterload
    B. end-diastolic volume
    C. blood pressure
    D. stroke volume

25. A person with a stroke volume of 70 ml and a heart rate of 80 has a cardiac output of
    A. 5600 ml
    B. 1500 ml
    C. 560 ml
    D. 150 ml

26. Preload is dependent upon
    A. arteriole vasoconstriction
    B. venous return
    C. stroke volume
    D. ventricular strength

27. The sympathetic nervous system innervates the heart via which receptors?
    A. Beta 1
    B. Beta 2
    C. Alpha 1
    D. Dopaminergic

28. The primary parasympathetic nerve that innervates the heart is the
    A. phrenic
    B. cardiac
    C. vagus
    D. acetylcholine

29. Which of the following could produce a parasympathetic response?
    A. Bearing down on the epiglottis
    B. Pressure on the carotid sinus
    C. Bladder distention
    D. All of the above

30. A positive inotropic drug increases
    A. heart rate
    B. conduction velocity
    C. contractile force
    D. refractoriness

31. A negative chronotropic drug decreases
    A. heart rate

    B. conduction velocity

    C. contractile force

    D. refractoriness

32. Specialized structures designed to speed conduction from one muscle fiber to the next are the

    A. syncytial tissues

    B. inotropic fibers

    C. intercalated discs

    D. autonomic cells

33. The ventricular syncytium occurs in an inferior to superior direction in order to

    A. direct blood to the aorta and pulmonary artery

    B. direct conduction to through the AV node

    C. enhance conduction velocity toward the atria

    D. avoid the vagus nerve

34. Which of the following is TRUE regarding the resting potential?

    A. Sodium is pumped into the cell

    B. Potassium is pumped out of the cell

    C. The inside of the cell is more negative than the outside

    D. The inside of the cell is more positive than the outside

35. Which of the following best characterizes the action potential?

    A. Potassium is actively pumped into the cell

    B. Sodium rapidly diffuses into the cell

    C. The inside of the cell becomes more negative

    D. The outside of the cell becomes more positive

36. The cells of the cardiac conductive system have

    A. automaticity

    B. excitability

    C. conductivity

    D. all of the above

37. The normal intrinsic firing rate of the SA node is

    A. 20-40 beats per minute

    B. 40-60 beats per minute

    C. 60-100 beats per minute

    D. none of the above

38. The normal intrinsic firing rate of the AV junction is

    A. 20-40 beats per minute

    B. 40-60 beats per minute

    C. 60-100 beats per minute

    D. none of the above

39. The normal intrinsic firing rate of the purkinje system is

    A. 20-40 beats per minute

    B. 40-60 beats per minute

    C. 60-100 beats per minute

    D. none of the above

40. According to Einthoven's Triangle, lead two is characterized by
A. left arm positive, right leg negative
B. left leg positive, right arm negative
C. right leg positive, left arm negative
D. right arm positive, left leg negative

41. Which of the following information can be obtained from a single lead ECG reading?
A. The presence of an infarct
B. Cardiac output
C. Chamber enlargement
D. Heart rate

42. On the vertical axis of a standard ECG graph paper, a deflection of two large boxes signifies
A. 1 mV of amplitude
B. 10 mV of amplitude
C. 0.4 seconds duration
D. 2.0 seconds duration

43. On the horizontal axis of a standard ECG graph paper, a deflection of one large box signifies
A. 1 mV of amplitude
B. 10 mV of amplitude
C. 0.2 seconds duration
D. 0.04 seconds duration

44. The P wave represents
A. atrial depolarization
B. ventricular depolarization
C. delay at the AV node
D. ventricular repolarization

45. The T wave represents
A. atrial depolarization
B. ventricular depolarization
C. delay at the AV node
D. ventricular repolarization

46. The QRS complex represents
A. atrial depolarization
B. ventricular depolarization
C. delay at the AV node
D. ventricular repolarization

47. The P-R interval represents
A. atrial depolarization
B. ventricular depolarization
C. delay at the AV node
D. ventricular repolarization

48. Which of the following is TRUE regarding the absolute refractory period?
A. The heart may depolarize
B. The heart cannot depolarize

C. It is represented by the T wave

D. It is the most vulnerable part of the cardiac cycle

49. Which of the following may produce artifact on the ECG?

A. Muscle tremors

B. Loose electrodes

C. 60 hertz interference

D. All of the above

50. Using the "Triplicate Method," how fast would the heart rate be if the R-R interval were three large boxes?

A. 60 beats per minute

B. 100 beats per minute

C. 150 beats per minute

D. 75 beats per minute

51. In normal sinus rhythm, the P waves should be

A. present

B. upright

C. alike

D. all of the above

52. The normal P-R interval is

A. < 0.12 seconds

B. 0.12—0.20 seconds

C. .04—0.1 seconds

D. none of the above

53. The normal QRS complex is

A. < 0.04 seconds

B. 0.12—0.20 seconds

C. 0.04—0.12 seconds

D. none of the above

54. Which of the following could cause a cardiac dysrhythmia?

A. Lateral wall myocardial infarction

B. Hyperkalemia

C. Hypoxia and acidosis

D. All of the above

55. Cardiac depolarization resulting from a focus other than a normal pacemaker cell is called

A. antegrade

B. retrograde

C. ectopic

D. reentry

SCENARIO Your patient is a 45-year-old male who experienced some chest discomfort while jogging. The pain is substernal and does not radiate. He has no previous medical history and takes no medications. The pain is somewhat relieved by rest. His BP is 150/88, pulse 96 and regular, respirations 18, skin warm and pink. His lungs are clear bilaterally and he has no other remarkable signs or symptoms. His EKG strip is as follows:

Figure 21-1

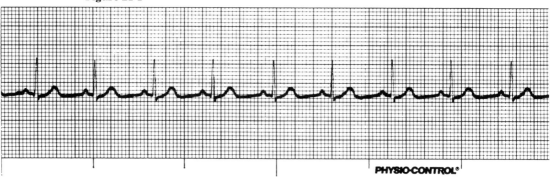

56. This patient's probable diagnosis is
   A. stable angina
   B. unstable angina
   C. pre-infarction angina
   D. Prinzmetals angina

57. His EKG strip is
   A. sinus tachycardia
   B. wandering atrial pacemaker
   C. premature atrial contractions
   D. normal sinus rhythm

58. Initial prehospital management of this patient should include oxygen and
   A. morphine IV
   B. nitroglycerine SL
   C. epinephrine SC
   D. atropine IV

SCENARIO Your patient is a 56-year-old female who complains of sudden onset of substernal chest pressure with no radiation while watching television. She denies any shortness of breath or nausea. She has a history of atherosclerotic heart disease and takes diltiazem. Her BP is 160/90, pulse is 110, respirations 16, skin warm and dry, lungs clear bilaterally. She has no other remarkable physical findings. Her EKG is as follows:

Figure 21-2

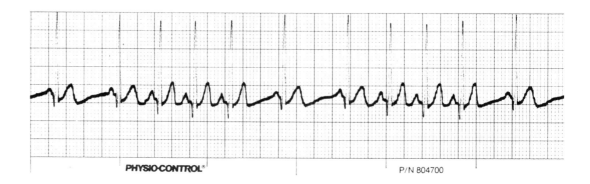

59. This patient is probably suffering from
   A. stable angina
   B. unstable angina
   C. cardiogenic shock
   D. Ludwig's angina

60. Her EKG strip is
   A. normal sinus rhythm
   B. premature atrial contraction
   C. wandering atrial pacemaker
   D. sinus dysrhythmia

61. The process by which fatty deposits collect within arterial walls is known as
   A. arteriosclerosis
   B. atherosclerosis
   C. arteriosclerotitis
   D. atheritis

62. Diltiazem is a drug in which class?
   A. Nitrate
   B. Beta blocker
   C. Calcium channel blocker
   D. Diuretic

SCENARIO Your patient is 65-year-old man who complains of sudden onset of substernal chest pain radiating to the neck and left shoulder. It began while eating one hour ago and has not subsided. He also complains of some shortness of breath, nausea, and dizzyness. He has a history of coronary artery disease and hypertension. He takes Procardia XL once-a-day. His BP is 180/80, pulse rate of 80 and irregular, respirations 26, lungs clear, skin warm and dry. His EKG strip is as follows:
Figure 21-3

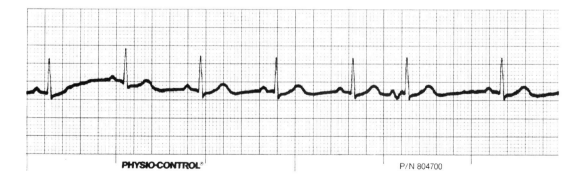

63. This patient is probably suffering from
   A. stable angina
   B. unstable angina

    C. acute myocardial infarction

    D. cardiogenic shock

64. His EKG strip is

    A. normal sinus rhythm

    B. premature atrial contraction

    C. wandering atrial pacemaker

    D. sinus dysrhythmia

65. Procardia XL is a drug in which class?

    A. Nitrate

    B. Beta blocker

    C. Calcium channel blocker

    D. Diuretic

66. Prehospital management of this patient includes

    A. high flow oxygen

    B. pain management

    C. reassurance

    D. all of the above

SCENARIO Your patient is a 25-year-old male with a congenital heart defect who presents with some chest pain and shortness of breath. He takes digoxin and claims that he often has problems. His BP is 170/80, pulse is 74 and irregular, respiratory rate of 18, skin warm and dry, lungs clear. His EKG is as follows:

Figure 21-4

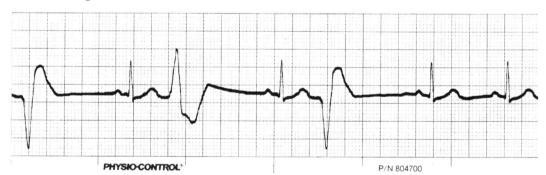

67. His EKG is

    A. premature atrial contractions

    B. ventricular bigeminy

    C. ventricular tachycardia

    D. premature ventricular contractions

68. Digoxin is a drug in which class?

    A. Nitrate

    B. Cardiac Glycoside

    C. Osmotic diuretic

    D. Calcium channel blocker

69. Prehospital management of this patient should include
    A. verapamil IV
    B. adenosine IV
    C. nifedipine IV
    D. lidocaine IV

SCENARIO Your patient is a 45-year-old female who complains of mild-to-moderate shortness of breath and some chest discomfort. She has a long history of cardiac problems and takes digoxin, Lasix, and Slo-K. Her BP is 180/80, pulse 94 and very irregular, respirations 20, skin cool and pink. She has bilateral crackles (rales) in the lower lobes. She has no peripheral edema or JVD. Her EKG is as follows:

Figure 21-5

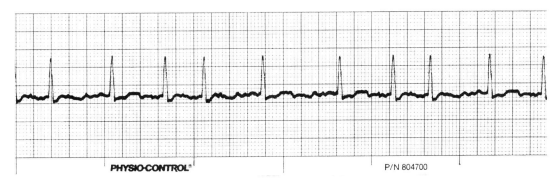

70. Your diagnosis of this patient is
    A. right heart failure
    B. left heart failure
    C. cardiogenic shock
    D. acute pulmonary edema

71. Her medications suggest she has
    A. abnormal cardiac dysrhythmias
    B. aortic valve problems
    C. corpulmonale
    D. congestive heart failure

72. Her EKG is
    A. wandering atrial pacemaker
    B. atrial flutter
    C. atrial fibrillation
    D. junctional rhythm

73. Prehospital pharmacological management of this patient should include oxygen and
    A. nitroglycerine, furosemide, morphine
    B. furosemide, albuterol, lidocaine

C. morphine, naloxone, furosemide

D. potassium, furosemide, morphine

SCENARIO   Your patient is an 80-year-old male who presents in severe respiratory distress, sitting bolt upright, gasping for each breath. He has a history of high blood pressure and breathing problems. He takes Inderal each day. His BP is 170/70, pulse is 72 and irregular, respirations 40 and extremely labored, skin warm and diaphoretic. Upon auscultation, you hear diffuse bilateral crackles and wheezing. He coughs up blood tinged sputum. His EKG is as follows:

Figure 21-6

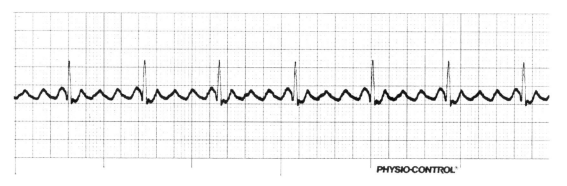

PHYSIO-CONTROL*

74. This patient is suffering from
A. acute pulmonary edema
B. corpulmonale
C. cardiogenic shock
D. aortic aneurysm

75. His EKG is
A. wandering atrial pacemaker
B. atrial flutter
C. atrial fibrillation
D. junctional rhythm

76. Inderal is a drug in which class?
A. Beta blocker
B. Nitrate
C. Calcium channel blocker
D. Cardiac glycoside

77. Which of the following is NOT a prehospital management goal for this patient?
A. Oxygenation
B. Preload increase
C. Diuresis
D. Coronary artery dilation

SCENARIO Your patient is a 57-year-old woman who lies unconscious on her living room floor. Her husband claims she "just collapsed after clutching her chest." She has a previous medical history and takes Cardizem. Her BP is 70 palpated, pulse is 140, respiratory rate 20 and shallow, skin cool, pale, and clammy, lungs congested, chemstrip is 130. Her EKG strip is as follows:

Figure 21-7

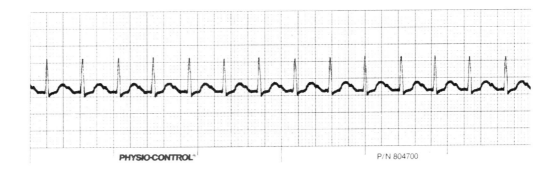

78. This patient is suffering from
    A. cardiogenic shock
    B. acute pulmonary edema
    C. right heart failure
    D. left heart failure

79. Her EKG is
    A. atrial fibrillation
    B. paroxysmal supraventricular tachycardia
    C. sinus tachycardia
    D. atrial flutter

80. The primary cause for this dysrhythmia is
    A. ectopic focus
    B. reentry focus
    C. compensatory mechanism
    D. parasympathetic stimulation

81. Cardizem is a drug in which class?
    A. Nitrate
    B. Cardiac glycoside
    C. Beta blocker
    D. Calcium channel blocker

82. Prehospital management of this patient includes all of the following **EXCEPT**
    A. dopamine IV
    B. oxygen
    C. IV fluid challenge
    D. positive pressure ventilation

SCENARIO   Your patient is a 78-year-old male who collapsed in the bathroom while moving his bowels. He sits slumped on the toilet, moaning, pale, and extremely diaphoretic. He has no history of cardiac problems and takes no medications. His BP is 70 palpated, pulse of 36, respirations 28 and shallow, lungs clear, chemstrip 120. His EKG is as follows:

Figure 21-8

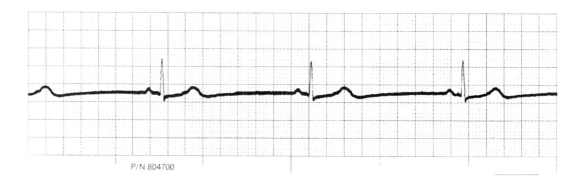

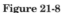

83. The most likely cause of this man's problem is
   A. hypoglycemia
   B. a vaso-vagal episode
   C. narcotic overdose
   D. sympathetic overstimulation

84. His EKG strip is
   A. junctional rhythm
   B. sinus arrhythmia
   C. sinus bradycardia
   D. idioventricular rhythm

85. The first prehospital treatment after oxygen is
   A. transcutaneous cardiac pacing
   B. adenosine IV
   C. epinephrine IV
   D. atropine IV

SCENARIO   Your patient is a 35-year-old female who developed heart palpitations while exercising. She complains of lightheadedness and some dizzyness. She denies any chest pain. She has a history of Wolff-Parkinson-White syndrome and takes Pronestyl. Her BP is 140/70, pulse of 190, respirations of 18, skin warm and dry, lungs clear bilaterally. Her EKG is as follows:

Figure 21-9

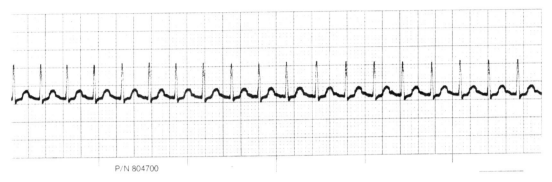

P/N 804700

86. This patient's rhythm is
   A. sinus tachycardia
   B. ventricular tachycardia
   C. supraventricular tachycardia
   D. atrial flutter

87. The probable cause of this dysrhythmia is
   A. ectopic focus in the ventricle
   B. reentry focus in the atria
   C. compensatory mechanism
   D. sympathetic stimulation

88. The initial treatment of this patient includes oxygen and
   A. immediate cardioversion
   B. immediate defibrillation
   C. vagal maneuvers
   D. verapamil IV

SCENARIO Your patient is a 67-year-old man who collapsed in the kitchen while cooking dinner. He presents on the floor, pale, clammy, moaning, with vomit around his mouth. His wife states he has no history and takes no medications. His BP is 70/30, pulse is 170 and weak, respirations are 28 and shallow, lungs are clear bilaterally, chemstrip 120. His EKG is as follows:

Figure 21-10

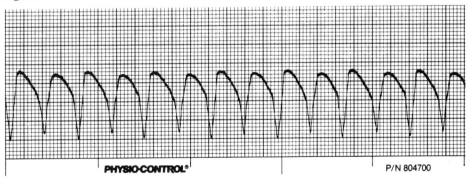

PHYSIO-CONTROL®   P/N 804700

89. His EKG is
  A. ventricular tachycardia
  B. SVT with aberrency
  C. ventricular fibrillation
  D. idioventricular rhythm

90. Initial management of this patient includes
  A. immediate synchronized cardioversion
  B. aggressive airway management
  C. diazepam IV
  D. all of the above

91. Which of the following drugs may be ordered for this patient?
  A. Atropine and epinephrine
  B. Adenosine and verapamil
  C. Naloxone and 50% dextrose
  D. Lidocaine and procainamide

SCENARIO Your patient is a 45-year-old male who complains of chest pain and shortness of breath. During your work-up he suddenly becomes unconscious and slumps over. His EKG changes are as follows:
Figure 21-11

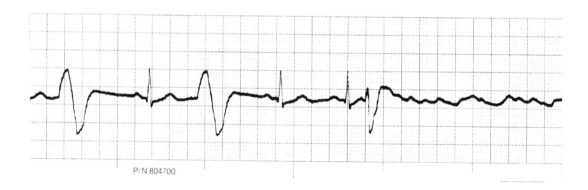

P/N 804700

92. This patient's new EKG is
  A. ventricular fibrillation
  B. ventricular tachycardia
  C. asystole
  D. idioventricular rhythm

93. Your first move is to
  A. defibrillate at 200 joules
  B. deliver a precordial thump
  C. begin CPR
  D. check your patient

94. All of the following will decrease intrathoracic resistance during defibrillation **EXCEPT**

    A. using electrode jelly

    B. using proper paddle pressure

    C. using proper paddle positioning

    D. waiting 3-5 minutes between defibrillation attempts

95. Pharmacological management of this patient includes which of the following drugs?

    A. Oxygen, epinephrine, atropine

    B. Oxygen, epinephrine, lidocaine, bretylium

    C. Oxygen, adenosine, verapamil, lidocaine

    D. Oxygen, epinephrine, isoproterenol, lidocaine

SCENARIO Your patient is a 99-year-old male found in cardiac arrest by his family. CPR was begun immediately and is ongoing upon your arrival. After a quick look, your patient is in the following rhythm. He is pulseless, apneic, unconscious.

Figure 21-12

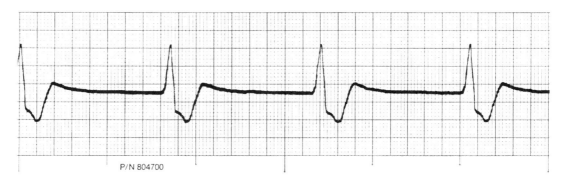

P/N 804700

96. This patient's rhythm is

    A. supraventricular tachycardia

    B. idioventricular rhythm

    C. ventricular tachycardia

    D. none of the above

97. This patient's condition is described as

    A. AV dissociation

    B. pulseless electrical activity

    C. complete heart block

    D. none of the above

98. Management of this patient includes all of the following EXCEPT

    A. CPR and intubation

    B. epinephrine and atropine IV

    C. defibrillation and lidocaine

    D. IV fluids

99. Causes for this condition include

    A. hypovolemia

    B. pericardial tamponade
    C. hypoxia and acidosis
    D. all of the above

SCENARIO   Your patient is a 65-year-old male complaining of malaise. He has no medical history and takes no medications. His BP is 120/70, pulse is 60 and irregular, respirations of 20, lungs clear, skin warm and dry. His EKG is as follows:

Figure 21-13

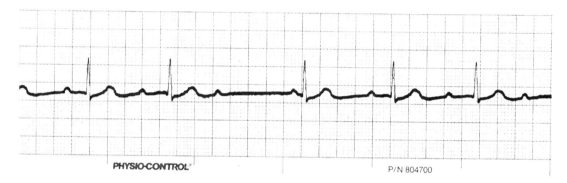

100.   This patient's rhythm is
    A. second degree AV block Type 2
    B. second degree AV block Type 1
    C. third degree AV block
    D. first degree AV block

101.   Prehospital management of this patient includes
    A. oxygen and monitoring only
    B. oxygen, atropine IV
    C. oxygen, transcutaneous pacing
    D. oxygen, atropine, transcutaneous pacing

SCENARIO   Your patient is an 89-year-old female who collapsed while shopping. No one is available to give you a history and she responds to deep pain only. Her BP is 70/30, pulse of 36, respirations 30 and shallow, skin pale and clammy, lungs clear bilaterally, chemstrip 100. Her EKG is as follows:

Figure 21-14

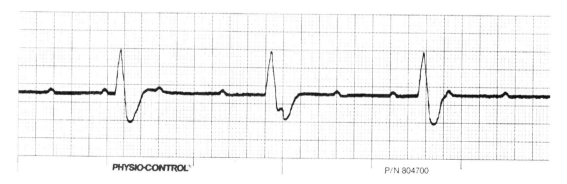

102. Her EKG is
   A. second degree AV block Type 2
   B. junctional escape rhythm
   C. third degree AV block
   D. ventricular excape rhythm

103. Prehospital management of this patient includes
   A. CPR and intubation
   B. atropine and transcutaneous pacing
   C. lidocaine and bretylium
   D. adenosine and verapamil

BCLS STANDARDS REVIEW

Activity	Infant (NB—1 yr)	Child (1—8 yrs)	Adult (> 8 yrs)
Compression depth			
Compression rate			
Comp / vent ratio			
FBO removal			

DRUG DOSE REVIEW

Drug	Adult	Pediatric
Nitroglycerine		
Morphine		
Furosemide		
Lidocaine		
Bretylium		
Adenosine		
Verapamil		
Epinephrine 1:10000		
Procainamide		
Magnesium		
Sodium Bicarbonate		
Norpepinephrine		
Isoproterenol		
Dopamine		
Dobutamine		

ANSWERS   **1. ANS—A**   *PEC—603*

The great vessels enter the heart through its base. The base is the top portion of the heart located at the level of the second rib. The great vessels include the inferior and superior vena cava, aorta, pulmonary arteries, and veins.

2. ANS—B   *PEC—603*

The inner-most layer of the heart which lines the chambers is the endocardium. It is the smoothest surface known to man.

3. ANS—A *PEC—603*

The thick middle layer of the heart wall containing the bulk of the muscle mass is the myocardium. The myocardium muscle cells are unique in that they physically resemble skeletal muscles, but they have electrical properties like smooth muscle.

4. ANS—C *PEC—603*

The visceral pericardium is the layer in contact with the heart muscle itself. The outermost lining of the heart, the epicardium, is contiguous with the visceral pericardium.

5. ANS—D *PEC—603*

Surrounding the heart is a protective sac, the pericardium. The pericardium consists of two layers, the visceral pericardium and the perital precardium. Situated between the two layers is pericardial fluid which acts as a lubricant during cardiac contraction.

6. ANS—C *PEC—604*

The heart contains four chambers. The two superior chambers which receive incoming blood are called atria. The larger inferior chambers are called ventricles.

7. ANS—D *PEC—606*

The only arteries in the body that carry oxygen-poor blood are the pulmonary arteries. These arteries carry blood from the right ventricle to the lungs for oxygenation.

8. ANS—B *PEC—606*

The only veins in the body that carry oxygen-rich blood are the pulmonary veins. These veins carry blood from the lungs back to the right atrium.

9. ANS—D *PEC—604*

The greatest muscle mass is found in the left ventricle. The left ventricle receives blood from the left atrium and pumps it out of heart into the aorta. The left side of the heart is the high-pressure side of the pump because of the high level of resistance present in the peripheral circulation.

10. ANS—B *PEC—604*

During systole the aortic and pulmonic valves are open allowing the heart to eject blood into the aorta and the pulmonary artery.

11. ANS—A *PEC—604*

During diastole, the mitral and tricuspid valves open to allow the atria to dump blood into the ventricles.

12. ANS—A *PEC—607*

The heart muscle itself is perfused by the coronary arteries. These vessels originate in the aorta just above the leaflets of the aortic valve and lie on the surface of the heart.

13. ANS—C *PEC—607*

Anastomoses between various branches of the coronary arteries allow for the development of collateral circulation. This is a protective mechanism which allows for an alternate path of blood flow in the event of vascular occlusion.

14. ANS—A   *PEC—607*

Deoxygenated blood is removed from the heart through the coronary veins. The coronary veins roughly respond to the coronary arteries and drain into the right atrium.

15. ANS—A   *PEC—608*

The innermost lining of the blood vessels, the tunic intima, is a single layer thick. This layer allows for rapid diffusion of blood gases to and from the tissues.

16. ANS—B   *PEC—608*

The muscular layer of the peripheral blood vessels is the tunica media consisting of elastic fibers and muscle. This layer gives blood vessels their strength and recoil which results from the difference in pressure inside and outside the cell.

17. ANS—D   *PEC—608*

Poiseuille's Law states that blood flow through a vessel is directly proportional to the fourth power of the vessel's diameter. This means that an increase or decrease in a blood vessel's size greatly influences the amount of blood flow through that vessel.

18. ANS—D   *PEC—608*

Gas exchange and cellular respiration occurs at the capillary level. The walls of the capillaries are a single cell layer thick which allows for exchange of gases, fluids, and nutrients between the vascular system and the tissues.

19. ANS—C   *PEC—608*

During diastole the ventricles fill with blood, the coronary arteries are perfused, and the artia contract sending blood down to the ventricles. The AV valves are open allowing this flow of blood.

20. ANS—D   *PEC—609*

Stroke volume is the amount of blood ejected by the heart in one contraction. Stroke volume is measured in milliliters. The average stroke volume is 60-100 milliliters although this capacity can increase significantly in a healthy heart.

21. ANS—C   *PEC—609*

Stroke volume is a reflection of three factors, preload, cardiac contractility, and afterload.

22. ANS—A   *PEC—609*

The pressure in the ventricle at the end diastole is referred to as preload. Preload influences the force of the next contraction. This is based on Starling's Law of the Heart which states that the more the myocardial muscle is stretched, up to a limit, the greater its force of contraction will be.

23. ANS—B   *PEC—610*

The resistance against which the heart must pump is called afterload. In general, the greater the resistance or afterload, the less the stroke volume. An increase in peripheral vascular resistance will decrease stroke volume. Conversely, a decrease in peripheral vascular resistance up to a point will increase stroke volume.

24. ANS—B *PEC—609*

Another name for preload is end-diastolic volume.

25. ANS—A *PEC—610*

Cardiac output is defined as the volume of blood pumped by the heart in one minute. It is a calculation of stroke volume times heart rate. A person with a stroke volume of 70 milliliters and heart rate of 80 beats per minute has a cardiac output therefore of 5600 milliliters.

26. ANS—B *PEC—609*

Preload represents the amount of blood or pressure in the ventricles prior to contraction. It is dependent upon venous return from the body.

27. ANS—A *PEC—611*

The sympathetic nervous system innervates the heart via the beta 1 receptors. When these receptors are stimulated, they cause the heart to increase its rate, force of contractions, and conductivity.

28. ANS—C *PEC—611*

The primary parasympathetic nerve that innervates the heart is the vagus nerve. The vagus nerve is also called cranial nerve #10 and arises from the base of the brain. The vagus nerve is responsible for regulating the heart's resting rate.

29. ANS—D *PEC—612*

The parasympathetic response can be produced by bearing down on the epiglottis, by putting pressure on the carotid sinus, or by bladder distention.

30. ANS—C *PEC—612*

The term inotropy refers to the strength of a muscular contraction of the heart. Therefore, a positive inotropic agent is one that increases the strength of a cardiac contraction.

31. ANS—A *PEC—612*

The term chronotrope refers to heart rate. A drug that is a negative chronotropic agent is one that suppresses the heart rate.

32. ANS—C *PEC—612*

Within the cardiac muscle fibers are special structures called intercalated disks. These disks connect cardiac muscle fibers and conduct electrical impulses quickly from one muscle fiber to the next.

33. ANS—A *PEC—612*

A syncytium is a group of cardiac muscle cells which physiologically function as a unit. The ventricular syncytium occurs in an inferior to superior direction in order to direct blood flow to the aorta and the pulmonary artery.

34. ANS—C *PEC—613*

The resting potential is the normal electrical state of cardiac cells. During this phase, sodium is actively pumped out of the cell membrane by a pump. This causes more negatively charged ions to remain inside the cell then positively charged ions which results in a difference of voltage across the cell membrane. Therefore, the inside of the cell is more negatively charged than the outside.

35. ANS—B *PEC—613*

During the action potential the membrane surrounding the cell changes instantaneously to allow sodium ions to rush into the cell bringing their positive charge.

Figure 21-15

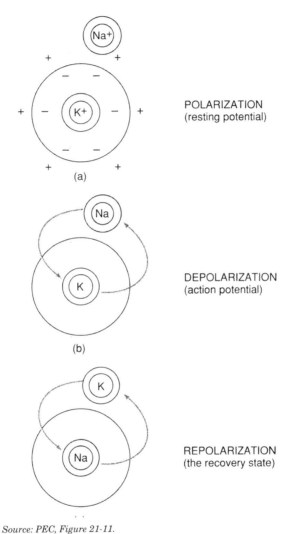

Source: PEC, Figure 21-11.

36. ANS—D *PEC—615*

The cells of the cardiac conductive system have several important properties. First, they have excitability. They can respond to electrical stimulus. Second, they have conductivity. They can conduct an electrical impulse from one cell to another, and third, they have automaticity, the ability to self-depolarize without an impulse from an outside source.

37. ANS—C *PEC—616*

The normal intrinsic firing rate of the SA node is 60-100 beats per minute.

38. ANS—B *PEC—616*

The normal intrinsic firing rate of the AV junction is 40-60 beats per minute.

39. ANS—A *PEC—616*

The normal intrinsic firing rate of the purkinje system is 20-40 beats per minute.

40. ANS—B *PEC—617*

According to Einthoven's Triangle, lead 2 is characterized by left-leg positive right-arm negative.

Figure 21-16

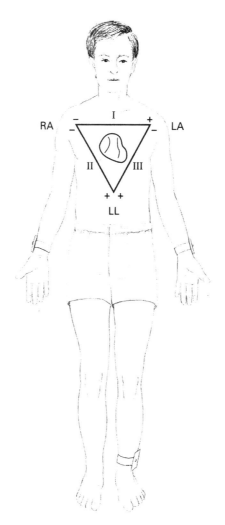

Source: PEC, Figure 21-13.

41. ANS—D *PEC—618*

Only a very limited amount of information can be obtained from a single lead ECG reading. You can tell how fast the heart is beating, how regular the heart beat is, and how long it takes to conduct the impulse through various parts of the heart. You cannot tell the presence or location of an infarct, chamber enlargement, or the quality or presence of pumping action.

42. ANS—A *PEC—619*

On the vertical axis of the standard ECG graph paper, a deflection of two large boxes signifies one milli volt of amplitude.

43. ANS—C *PEC—619*

On the horizontal axis of the standard ECG graph paper, a deflection of one large box signifies 0.2 seconds duration.

44. ANS—A *PEC—619*

The P wave represents each atrial depolarization.

Figure 21-17

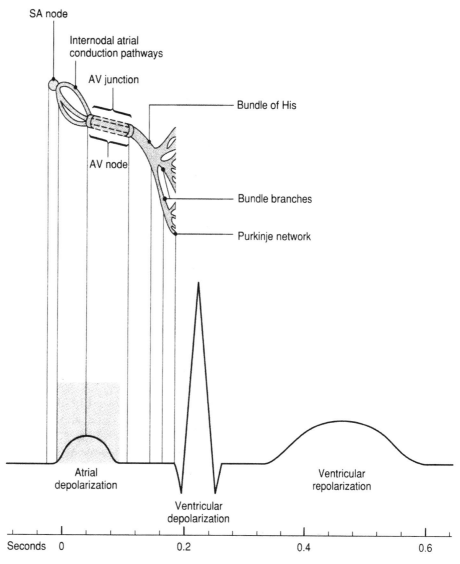

Source: PEC, Figure 21-16.

45. ANS—D *PEC—620*

The T wave represents ventricular repolarization.

46. ANS—B *PEC—620*

The QRS complex represents ventricular depolarization.

47. ANS—C *PEC—620*

The P-R interval represents delay at the AV node. The normal P-R interval is 0.12—0.20 seconds.

48. ANS—B   *PEC—625*

The absolute refractory period represents the period of the cardiac cycle when stimulation will not produce any depolarization whatsoever. This usually lasts from the beginning of the QRS complex to the tip of the T wave.

Figure 21-18

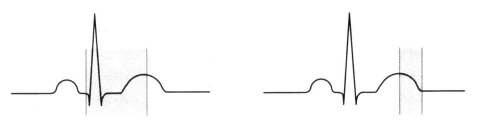

Absolute Refractory Period   Relative Refractory Period

Source: PEC, Figure 21-25.

49. ANS—D   *PEC—625*

Artifacts are deflections produced by factors other than the heart's electrical activity. Common causes of artifacts include muscle tremors, shivering, patient movement, loose electrodes, 60 Hz interference, and machine malfunction.

50. ANS—B   *PEC—626*

Using the triplicate method, if the R-R interval were three large boxes, the rate would be 100. First locate an R wave that falls on a dark line bordering a large box on the graph paper, then assign numbers corresponding to the heart rate to the next six dark lines to the right. The order is 300, 150, 100, 75, 60, and 50. The number corresponding to the dark line closest to the peak of the next R wave is a rough estimate of the heart rate.

51. ANS—D   *PEC—627*

In normal sinus rhythm the P wave should be present, it should be upright in lead 2, and they should all look alike.

52. ANS—B   *PEC—627*

The normal P-R interval is 0.12 to 0.20 seconds.

53. ANS—C   *PEC—627*

The normal QRS complex is 0.04 to 0.12 seconds.

54. ANS—D   *PEC—627*

Dysrhythmias are deviations from the normal electrical rhythm of the heart and can be caused by a number of situations: myocardial ischemia and infarction, electrolyte imbalances such as hyperkalemia, and blood gas abnormalities including hypoxia and an abnormal pH.

55. ANS—C   *PEC—628*

Cardiac depolarization resulting from depolarization from cells in the heart that are not a part of the heart's normal pacemaker system are known as ectopic beats.

56. ANS—A   *PEC—689*

Stable angina occurs during activity when oxygen demands of the heart are increased. Angina can be of relatively short duration, 3-5 minutes, or prolonged lasting 15 minutes or more. The pain is often relieved by rest, nitroglycerin, or oxygen.

57. ANS—D *PEC—627*

Sinus rhythm is the standard heart beat. It is distinguished by the following features: rate 60-100 beats per minute; P to P and R to R rhythms are regular; P waves are normal in shape, upright, and appear only before each QRS complex. The P-R interval lasts 0.12 to 0.20 seconds and is constant. The QRS complex looks normal and has a duration less than 0.12 seconds.

58. ANS—B *PEC—627*

Initial prehospital management of this patient should include oxygen and nitroglycerin sublingually. Nitroglycerin decreases myocardial work and dilates the coronary arteries.

59. ANS—B *PEC—689*

Unstable angina occurs at rest. Because this condition often indicates severe atherosclerotic heart disease, it's also called pre-infarction angina.

60. ANS—D *PEC—689*

Sinus dysrhythmia is often a normal finding and is sometimes related to the respiratory cycle and changes in intrathoracic pressure. It can also be caused by enhanced vagal tone. Identifying features of sinus dysrhythmia include an irregular rhythm. In all other ways it is identical to normal sinus rhythm.

61. ANS—B *PEC—688*

The major underlying factor in many cardiovascular emergencies is atherosclerosis. Atherosclerosis is a progressive, degenerative disease of the medium and large arteries. It results from the deposition of fats under the tunica intima layer of the involved vessels.

62. ANS—C *PEC—712*

Diltiazem (Cardizem) is a calcium channel blocker, a relatively new class of medication. These agents are being used increasingly for angina pectoris, dysrhythmias, hypertension, and other cardiovascular problems. They work by inhibiting calcium from entering the cells.

63. ANS—C *PEC—690*

Acute myocardial infarction is the death of a portion of the heart muscle from prolonged deprivation of arterial blood supply. It can also occur when the oxygen demand of the heart exceeds its supply for an extended period of time. It is most often associated with atherosclerotic heart disease.

64. ANS—B *PEC—641*

Premature atrial contractions result from a single electrical impulse originating in the atria outside the SA node which in turn causes a premature depolarization of the heart before the next expected sinus beat. Identifying features of a PAC include an early beat with a normal looking P wave and normal looking QRS.

65. ANS—C *PEC -712*

Nifedipine (Procardia) is a calcium channel blocker.

66. ANS—D *PEC—692*

Prehospital management of a patient with acute myocardial infarction includes preventing pain and apprehension by reassuring the patient, administering high-flow oxygen, and managing pain with nitroglycerin and morphine.

67. ANS—D *PEC—662*

Premature ventricular contraction is a single ectopic impulse arising from an irritable focus in either ventricle that occurs earlier than the next expected beat. It may result from increased automaticity in the ectopic cell or a reentry mechanism. Identifying features of a PVC are a wide bizarre QRS complex, and an early beat without a P wave.

68. ANS—B *PEC—712*

Digoxin is a cardiac glycoside. It increases the force of cardiac contraction and cardiac output and slows impulse conduction through the AV node decreasing the ventricular response to certain super-ventricular dysrhythmias, such as atrial fibrillation, atrial flutter, and PSVT. It is also used in the treatment of heart failure and the dysrhythmias mentioned above.

69. ANS—D *PEC—663*

Prehospital management of malignant PVCs includes administration of lidocaine. Administer lidocaine at a dose of 1.0—1.5 mg/kg of body weight. Give an additional lidocaine bolus of 0.5—0.75 mg/kg every 5 minutes if necessary until a total of 3.0 mg/kg of the drug has been given. If the PVCs are effectively suppressed, start a lidocaine drip beginning at a rate of 2-4 mg/min.

70. ANS—B *PEC—694*

Left ventricular failure occurs when the left ventricle fails as an effective forward pump causing back pressure of blood into the pump pulmonary circulation often resulting in pulmonary edema. The patient with left heart failure usually presents with bilateral rales in the lower lobes and shortness of breath.

71. ANS—D *PEC—711*

A patient with a history of congestive heart failure may take digoxin to increase cardiac output by increasing the force of contraction of the left ventricle. He may take a diuretic to decrease venous return and stimulate the kidneys to produce more urine and a potassium supplement such as slow- K to replenish potassium loss through excessive diuresis.

72. ANS—C *PEC—649*

Atrial fibrillation is a dysrhythmia that results from multiple areas of re-entry within the atria or from multiple ectopic foci bombarding an AV node. Identifying features of atrial fibrillation include a grossly irregular rhythm and no discernible P waves.

73. ANS—A *PEC—696*

The goals of prehospital management of a patient in left ventricular failure includes decreasing venous return to the heart, decreasing myocardial oxygen demands, and improving ventilation and oxygenation. Pharmacologically we do this by administering nitroglycerin, furrosemide, and morphine.

74. ANS—A *PEC—694*

Acute pulmonary edema is the most serious complication of left ventricular failure when the lungs are literally bombarded with fluid. The fluid leaks out of the capillary beds into the interstitial spaces.

75. ANS—B *PEC—647*

Atrial flutter results from a rapid atrial re-entry circuit and an AV node that cannot handle all impulses through to the ventricles. Identifying features of atrial flutter include the absence of P waves and the presence of flutter waves at a rate of 250-350 per minute. The flutter waves resemble a saw tooth or picket fence pattern.

76. ANS—A *PEC—712*

Beta blockers are frequently used to control dysrhythmias, high blood pressure, and angina. Many beta blockers such as propranolol (Inderal) are non-selective while others are selective for beta 1 or beta 2 receptors.

77. ANS—B *PEC—696*

Prehospital management of a patient in acute pulmonary edema includes decreasing venous return of the heart, decreasing myocardial oxygen demands, and improving ventilation and oxygenation.

78. ANS—A *PEC—699*

Cardiogenic shock is the most severe form of pump failure. It occurs when left ventricular function is so compromised that the heart cannot meet the metabolic demands of the body and compensatory mechanisms are exhausted.

79. ANS—C *PEC—633*

Sinus tachycardia results from an increase in the rate of SA node discharge. Tachycardia is identical to normal sinus rhythm except that the rate is greater than 100.

80. ANS—C *PEC—633*

Sinus tachycardia is often a benign process. In some cases it is a compensatory mechanism for decreased stroke volume.

81. ANS—D *PEC—712*

Diltiazem (Cardizem) is a calcium channel blocker. Calcium channel blockers are used increasingly for angina, dysrhythmias, hypertension, and other cardiovascular problems.

82. ANS—C *PEC—699*

Prehospital management of the patient in cardiogenic shock is difficult. Even when the best technology is available, mortality rates approach 80-90 percent. Prehospital management should include rapid transport, high-flow oxygen, and starting a dopamine drip.

83. ANS—B *PEC—631*

The most common cause of this man's syncope is a vaso-vagal episode.

84. ANS—C *PEC—641*

Sinus bradycardia results from slowing of the SA node. It can result from increased parasympathetic tone, SA node disease, or drug effects.

85. ANS—D *PEC—631*

Treatment of sinus bradycardia is unnecessary unless hypotension or ventricular irritability is present. If treatment is required, administer 0.5 mg bolus of atropine sulfate. This can be repeated every 3-5 minutes until a satisfactory rate has been obtained or 0.04 mg/kg of the drug has been given.

86. ANS—C   *PEC—643*

Supraventricular tachycardia occurs when rapid atrial depolarization overrides the SA node. It often occurs with a sudden onset, may last minutes to hours.

87. ANS—B   *PEC—643*

Supraventricular tachycardia may be caused by increased automaticity of a single atrial focus or by re-entry phenomena at the AV node.

88. ANS—C   *PEC—645*

Initial treatment of a patient in supraventricular tachycardia with stable vital signs includes oxygen and performing vagal maneuvers such as Valsalva or carotid sinus massage.

89. ANS—A   *PEC—665*

Ventricular tachycardia is a rhythm that consists of three or more ventricular complexes in succession at a rate of 100 beats per minute or more. This rhythm overrides the normal pacemaker of the heart.

90. ANS—A   *PEC—666*

Initial management of this patient includes immediate synchronized cardioversion.

91. ANS—D   *PEC—666*

Pharmacological management of this patient may include lidocaine and procainamide.

92. ANS—A   *PEC—669*

Ventricular fibrillation is a chaotic ventricular rhythm usually resulting from the presence of many re-entry circuits within the ventricles. There is no ventricular depolarization or contraction.

93. ANS—D   *PEC—669*

The initial management of this patient is to check him clinically. Always correlate your patient's pulse with what you see on the ECG. In this case, a disconnected lead or faulty monitor could produce this ECG pattern. If you cannot detect a pulse, consider the rhythm ventricular fibrillation.

94. ANS—D   *PEC—716*

Reducing intrathoracic resistance is an important factor in a successful defibrillation. Using electrode jelly, proper paddle positioning and pressure, and delivering successive countershocks as quickly as possible will all decrease intrathoracic resistance.

95. ANS—B   *PEC—702*

Pharmacological management of the patient with ventricular fibrillation includes oxygen, epinephrine, lidocaine, and bretylium.

96. ANS—B   *PEC—661*

Ventricular escape rhythm or idioventricular rhythm results when either impulses from the higher pacemakers fail to reach the ventricles or the rate of discharge of higher pacemakers become less than that of the ventricles, normally 15-45 beats per minute.

97. ANS—B *PEC—661*

When a patient with a rhythm has no associated pulse, this is known as pulseless electrical activity.

98. ANS—C *PEC—704*

Management of a patient in idioventricular rhythm with pulses electrical activity includes CPR; airway management and oxygenation, including intubation; epinephrine and atropine IV; and rapid IV fluid administration.

99. ANS—D *PEC—661*

Common causes for pulseless electrical activity include hypovolemia, hypoxia, acidosis, and cardiac tamponade.

100. ANS—B *PEC—677*

Second degree AV block type 1 (Wenkebach phenomenon) is an intermittent block at the level of the AV node. It produces a characteristic cyclic pattern in which the P-R intervals become progressively longer until an impulse is blocked or not conducted through the AV node. This cycle is repetitive. Identifying features of second degree AV block type 1 is a P-R interval that progressively lengthens until a QRS complex is dropped.

101. ANS—A *PEC—677*

There is generally no treatment other than observation for patients in second degree AV block type 1.

102. ANS—C *PEC—681*

Third degree block, or complete heart block, is the absence of conduction between the atria and the ventricles resulting from complete electrical block at or below the AV node. The atria and ventricles subsequently pace the heart independent of each other.

103. ANS—B *PEC—681*

Third degree heart block can severely compromise cardiac output because of decreased heart rate and the loss of coordinated atrial kick. The prehospital management of this patient would include parasympathetic blockers such as atropine and transcutaneous external pacing.

BCLS STANDARDS REVIEW

Activity	Infant (NB—1 yr)	Child (1—8 yrs)	Adult (> 8 yrs)
Compression depth	1/2—1 inch	1—1 1/2 inch	1 1/2—2 inches
Compression rate	≥100 / min	80—100 / min	80 m—100 / min
Comp / vent ratio	5 / 1	5 / 1	15 / 2, 5 / 1

DRUG DOSE REVIEW

Drug	Adult	Pediatric
Nitroglycerine	0.4 mg SL	-
Morphine	2-5 mg IV	-
Furosemide	20-80 mg IV	-
Lidocaine	1.0—1.5 mg/kg IV	1 mg/kg IV
Bretylium	5 mg/kg IV	5 mg/kg IV
Adenosine	6 mg IV	0.1—0.2 mg/kg IV
Verapamil	2.5-5 mg IV	-
Epinephrine 1:10000	1.0 mg IV	0.01 mg/kg IV/IO
Procainamide	20 mg/min	-
Magnesium	1-2 grams IV	-
Sodium Bicarbonate	1 mEq/kg IV	1 mEq/kg IV
Norpepinephrine	0.5-1.0 mcg/min	-
Isoproterenol	2-10 mcg/min	-
Dopamine	5 mcg/kg/min	2-20 mcg/kg/min
Dobutamine	2-20 mcg/kg/min	2-20 mcg/kg/min

CHAPTER 22

Endocrine Emergencies

QUESTIONS

1. Chemical substances released by a gland that controls or affects other glands or body systems are called
   A. endocrines
   B. hormones
   C. polypeptides
   D. ketones

2. The master gland whose function is to control the other endocrine glands is the
   A. pituitary
   B. thyroid
   C. adrenal
   D. endocrine

3. The hormone produced by the posterior pituitary gland that helps control fluid regulation is
   A. antidiuretic hormone
   B. vasopressin
   C. prolactin
   D. A and B

4. Oxytocin, when released, causes
   A. uterine contractions
   B. egg implantation in the uterus

   C. feminization
   D. maturation of the egg

5. You can suppress preterm labor by administering a fluid bolus because
   A. the mother is usually dehydrated
   B. oxytocin release is inhibited
   C. the fluid increase fools the thyroid gland
   D. less ACTH is secreted

6. Graves disease, characterized by insomnia, tachycardia, hypertension, and fatigue, is the result of
   A. hyponatremia
   B. hyperadrenalism
   C. hyperthyroidism
   D. hypocalcemia

7. Myxedema, characterized by facial bloating, weakness, altered mental status, and oily skin is caused by
   A. hypothyroidism
   B. hyperadrenalism
   C. hypernatremia
   D. hypocalcemia

8. The parathyroid glands are responsible for regulating blood levels of
   A. glucose
   B. calcium
   C. insulin
   D. ADH

9. Which of the following hormones stimulates the liver to transform its glycogen stores into glucose for immediate use?
   A. Prolactin
   B. Glucagon
   C. Insulin
   D. Somatostatin

10. Which of the following hormones is **NOT** produced by the islets of Langerhans?
    A. Glucagon
    B. Somatostatin
    C. Prolactin
    D. Insulin

11. Insulin is necessary to
    A. facilitate transport of glucose into the cells
    B. produce glucose from muscle tissue
    C. enhance glycogen formation in the liver
    D. promote gluconeogenesis

12. Cathecholamines are released by the
    A. adrenal medulla

    B. adrenal cortex

    C. islets of Langerhans

    D. pancreas

13. The adrenal cortex releases

    A. corticosteroids

    B. anti-inflammatory agents

    C. mineralocorticoids

    D. all of the above

14. Oversecretion by the adrenal cortex results in a condition known as

    A. Grave's disease

    B. myxedema

    C. diabetes mellitus

    D. Cushing's disease

15. The ovaries are responsible for all of the following except

    A. manufacturing estrogen and progesterone

    B. preparing the uterus for egg implantation

    C. secreting testosterone

    D. female sexual development

16. The testes are controlled by the hormone(s)

    A. estrogen and progesterone

    B. FSH and LH

    C. TSH and GH

    D. prolactin

17. Which of the following is **NOT** a characteristic of diabetes mellitus?

    A. Ketone production

    B. Excessive insulin production

    C. Osmotic diuresis

    D. Associated heart and kidney disease

18. Diabetic ketoacidosis is a direct result of

    A. the cells burning inefficient fuels

    B. the pancreas secreting excessive insulin

    C. the kidneys reabsorbing glucose

    D. rapid, deep respirations

19. Insulin shock is a direct result of

    A. insufficient insulin levels

    B. insufficient blood glucose levels

    C. hyperglycemia

    D. not taking enough insulin

20. Non-ketotic hyperosmolar coma differs from DKA in that

    A. the pancreas produces some insulin

    B. ketones are eliminated by the kidneys

    C. osmotic diuresis does not occur

    D. blood glucose levels do not rise greatly

SCENARIO Your patient is a 45-year-old male who lies unconscious in bed. His daughter states that he has a long history of diabetes and takes insulin daily. He lives alone and hasn't been seen for a few days. He has no other history. His heart rate is 100; blood pressure 90/60; respiratory rate 40 and deep with a fruity odor; lungs clear, skin warm and dry; chemstrip is 380. He has vomited twice prior to your arrival.

21. This patient is most likely suffering from
    A. hypoglycemia
    B. insulin shock
    C. hyperglycemia
    D. non-ketotic hyperosmolar coma

22. His problem probably resulted from
    A. taking his insulin and not eating enough
    B. not taking his insulin
    C. taking his insulin and overeating
    D. recent illness

23. His hypotension and dehydrated look result from
    A. osmotic diuresis
    B. overproduction of ketones
    C. increased insulin levels
    D. increased ADH release

24. His respiratory pattern is known as
    A. Cheyne-Stokes
    B. Kussmaul's
    C. Graves
    D. Biot's

25. This respiratory pattern occurs as the body attempts to
    A. increase insulin production
    B. correct metabolic acidosis
    C. decrease hypoxia from insulin shock
    D. produce more ketonic acids

26. The fruity breath results from _____ in the expired air.
    A. glucose
    B. insulin
    C. ketones
    D. glucagon

27. His chemstrip reads 380 because
    A. he cannot transport glucose into his cells
    B. he cannot transform glycogen into glucose
    C. he is hypoglycemic
    D. he is in insulin shock

28. Classic early signs of this disease include all of the following except
    A. polydipsia

    B. polyurea
    C. polyphagia
    D. polyphasia

29. Emergency prehospital treatment for this patient includes
    A. crystalloid fluid infusion
    B. 50% dextrose IV
    C. glucagon IM
    D. naloxone IV

SCENARIO Your patient is a 39-year-old female who collapsed in a supermarket and lies unconscious on the floor. She is alone and no one is available to provide you with a history. She has no medications in her purse, except for some Glucotabs. She is wearing a bracelet that states she is diabetic. Her heart rate is 110; her blood pressure is 100/70; her respiratory rate is 28 and shallow; skin cool and clammy; lungs clear; chemstrip 40.

30. This patient is most likely suffering from
    A. hypoglycemia
    B. insulin shock
    C. hyperglycemia
    D. A and B

31. This patient's condition could have resulted from any of the following except
    A. taking her insulin, not eating enough
    B. not taking her insulin
    C. too much exercise/activity
    D. recent illness

32. Her unconsciousness is due to
    A. cerebral hypoxia
    B. cerebral hypoglycemia
    C. ketoacidosis
    D. osmotic diuresis

33. Prehospital management of this patient includes
    A. insulin SC
    B. 250 ml of Lactated Ringer's
    C. 50% dextrose IV
    D. naloxone IV

34. If an accurate chemstrip cannot be obtained, management should include all of the following except
    A. thiamine IV
    B. 50% dextrose IV
    C. insulin SC
    D. naloxone IV

DRUG DOSE REVIEW

Drug	Adult	Pediatric
50% Dextrose		
Glucagon		
Thiamine		

ANSWERS

1. ANS—B   *PEC—726*

Hormones are chemical substances released by glands that control or affect other glands or body systems. Endocrine glands secrete hormones directly into the bloodstream. Exocrine glands transport their hormones to target tissues via ducts. Emergencies are usually caused by the underproduction or overproduction of hormones.

2. ANS—A   *PEC—726*

The pituitary gland is known as the "master gland." It's primary function is to regulate the other endocrine glands. It is located at the base of the brain and is very well protected.

3. ANS—D   *PEC—727*

The posterior pituitary gland produces two hormones: oxytocin and antidiuretic hormone (ADH). ADH, also called "vasopressin", stimulates the kidneys to retain water by reabsorbing sodium to compensate for fluid volume losses. After fluid levels stabilize, the pituitary gland inhibits ADH secretion.

4. ANS—A   *PEC—727*

Oxytocin stimulates contraction of the uterine musculature and milk "let down" from the breast. Oxytocin is the naturally occuring form of the drug pitocin. In the hospital it is used to induce labor by contracting the uterus. In the field, paramedics administer oxytocin to control postpartum hemorrhage.

5. ANS—B   *PEC—728*

Oxytocin and ADH have an interesting relationship. They are both secreted by the posterior pituitary gland. Preterm labor, also called "Braxton-Hicks" labor is caused by premature uterine contractions. By administering a fluid bolus, intravascular fluid volume is increased, signalling the brain to stop secreting ADH. Since oxytocin is secreted by the same area of the pituitary, it's release is also inhibited. By stopping oxytocin release, the uterine contractions subside and the labor pains stop.

6. ANS—C   *PEC—728*

The thyroid gland controls the rate of metabolism. Overproduction of thyroid hormones causes Grave's disease. It is characterized by insomnia, fatigue, tachycardia, hypertension, heat intolerance, and weight loss. In severe cases, thyrotoxicosis may occur—a medical emergency.

7. ANS—A   *PEC—728*

Inadequate levels of thyroid hormones result in myxedema. This disorder includes facial bloating, weakness, cold intolerance, oily skin and hair, altered mental states, and a 50% mortality. People with hypothyroidism take a synthetic thyroid hormone.

8. ANS—B   *PEC—728*

The parathyroid glands produce a hormone called parathyroid hormone which causes increases in the blood level of calcium. These glands are located in the neck near the thyroid.

9. ANS—B   *PEC—729*

Glucagon stimulates the liver to transform its glycogen stores into glucose for immediate use. It also stimulates the liver to manufacture glucose from other sustances in a process called gluconeogenesis. Glucagon raises the blood levels of glucose.

10. ANS—C   *PEC—729*

The islets of Langerhans are specialized tissues within the pancreas that contain three types of hormone-secreting cells: alpha cells, beta cells, and delta cells. Alpha cells secrete glucagon; beta cells secrete insulin; and delta cells secrete somatostatin.

11. ANS—A   *PEC—729*

Insulin is a hormone secreted by the beta cells of the islets of Langerhans. It is antagonistic to glucagon and causes blood levels of glucose to decrease. It combines with insulin receptors on the cell membrane and allows glucose to enter the cell. It is an absolute necessity for survival.

12. ANS—A   *PEC—729*

The catecholamines, epinephrine and norepinephrine, are secreted by the adrenal glands, specifically the adrenal medulla. These hormones stimulate the sympathetic nervous system to prepare the body for extreme stressors.

13. ANS—D   *PEC—729*

The adrenal cortex secretes three classes of hormones: glucocorticoids, mineralocorticoids, and androgenic hormones. Like the catecholamines, these steroidal hormones respond to body stressors by raising blood glucose levels and performing anti-inflammatory and immune supression duties.

14. ANS—D   *PEC—730*

Prolonged secretion of adrenal cortex hormones may result in Cushing's disease. This disease is characterized by increased blood sugar levels, unusual body fat distribution, and rapid mood swings. If electrolyte imbalances occur as a result of this disease, serious complications may arise, including cardiac dysrhythmias, coma, and death. This condition is usually caused by a tumor.

15. ANS—C   *PEC—730*

The ovaries are the female sex glands located adjacent to the uterus. They produce eggs for reproduction and manufacture estrogen and progesterone which aid in sexual development and in preparing the uterus for egg implantation. The ovaries are controlled by the anterior pituitary hormones FSH (follicle stimulating hormone) and LH (luteinizing hormone).

16. ANS—B *PEC—730*

The testes are the male sex glands located in the scrotum. They produce sperm for reproduction and manufacture testosterone which promotes male growth and masculinization. The testes are also controlled by the anterior pituitary hormones FSH (follicle stimulating hormone) and LH (luteinizing hormone).

17. ANS—B *PEC—730*

Diabetes mellitus is a disease characterized by decreased insulin production by the beta cells of the islets of Langerhans of the pancreas. Insulin facilitates glucose transport into the cells. As the body cells become starved for glucose, they use other sources of energy, resulting in ketone production. Increased blood glucose levels cause an osmotic gradient resulting in a water shift into the vascular compartment. This, in turn, causes glucose to be spilled into the urine, taking water with it. The diabetic is at risk for heart disease, kidney failure, and blindness.

18. ANS—A *PEC—731*

Diabetic ketoacidosis is a direct result of the cells using other sources of energy, such as fats. This inefficient fuel produces many by-products, such as ketones and other organic acids. If enough ketones are produced, metabolic acidosis and coma may ensue.

19. ANS—B *PEC—732*

Insulin shock (hypoglycemia) is a result of insufficient glucose to meet tissue demands. Usually this occurs as a result of taking injected insulin and not eating enough to feed the tissues. The insulin transports all available glucose into the cells leaving very low blood levels. Untreated, the patient may sustain brain injury since it receives its energy from glucose metabolism. Hypoglycemia is a true emergency.

20. ANS—A *PEC—731*

Non-ketotic hyperosmolar coma differs from diabetic coma. These patients produce enough insulin to feed the cells, but not enough to maintain normal blood glucose levels. Their glucose can reach extremely high levels, causing a tremendous osmotic gradient and dehydration. Ketones are not produced because glucose is burned as fuel in the cells.

21. ANS—C *PEC—732*

This patient is most likely suffering from diabetic ketoacidosis (DKA) or hyperglycemia. The history (positive for diabetes); onset (slow); chemstrip (high); respirations (rapid and deep); and skin condition (warm and dry) are all classic signs.

22. ANS—B *PEC—732*

Hyperglycemia most often results from not taking sufficient amounts of prescribed insulin. Without this messenger, glucose cannot enter the cells.

23. ANS—A *PEC—732*

Increased blood glucose levels cause an osmotic gradient. This gradient draws interstitial water into the intravascular compartment resulting in glucose spillage into the urine. As water follows glucose, patients become dehydrated. If enough fluid is lost, hypotension and tachycardia follow.

24. ANS—B *PEC—732*

Kussmaul's respirations are characterized by rapid, deep breathing. It represents the body's attempt to increase minute volume. The pattern is identified as below:

Figure 22-1

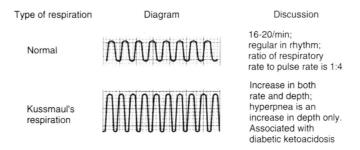

Source: PEC, Figure 22-3.

25. ANS—B *PEC—732*

Kussmaul's respirations are the body's attempt to compensate for the metabolic acidosis caused by excessive ketone production. As the buffer system changes metabolic acids (ketones) to respiratory acids (carbon dioxide), the respiratory system eliminates the excess by increasing minute volume ventilation. Minute volume is increased by breathing faster and deeper than normal.

26. ANS—C *PEC—732*

When ketones are eliminated through the respiratory tract, the patient will exhibit a fruity, or acetone, breath odor.

27. ANS—A *PEC—732*

Because this patient cannot transport glucose into his cells, blood levels rise dramatically.

28. ANS—D *PEC—732*

The early signs of diabetes include polyurea (frequent urination from osmotic diuresis), polydipsia (excessive thirst from the dehydration), and polyphagia (excessive hunger from the cells being starved of glucose).

29. ANS—A *PEC—732*

If blood glucose levels can be accurately determined to be high and the patient exhibits the signs and symptoms of DKA, a crystalloid infusion should be administered to reverse the dehydration and hypotension. A red top can be drawn to obtain baseline glucose levels. If allowed, insulin may be administered in the field.

30. ANS—D *PEC—734*

Your patient is most likely suffering from insulin shock (hypoglycemia). Her history (Medic-alert bracelet and Glucotabs); level of consciousness (altered); and chemstrip (low) all strongly suggest hypoglycemia. An altered level of consciousness, low chemstrip, and improvement following dextrose therapy is known as "Whipple's Triad."

31. ANS—B *PEC—734*

Hypoglycemia may result from taking too much insulin, not eating enough, excessive exercise, or illness.

32. ANS—B   *PEC—734*

This patient has no available glucose for brain metabolism. The brain is a very greedy organ, demanding a constant supply of oxygen and glucose. Withhold either from the brain for an extended period of time and death may result.

33. ANS—C   *PEC—734*

Prehospital treatment of this patient includes a rapid bolus of 25 grams of 50% dextrose IV. A red top can be drawn to determine baseline blood levels.

34. ANS—C   *PEC—734*

If blood glucose levels cannot be determined, a rapid bolus of 25 grams of 50% dextrose IV followed by 100 mg of thiamine IV and 1-2 mg of naloxone should be administered.

DRUG DOSE REVIEW

Drug	Adult	Pediatric
50% Dextrose	25 grams IV	0.5-1 gm/kg IV
Glucagon	0.5-1 mg IM	0.1 mg/kg IM
Thiamine	100 mg IV	rarely used

CHAPTER 23

Nervous System
Emergencies

QUESTIONS

1. The central nervous system consists of the
   A. sympathetic and parasympathetic branches
   B. cranial nerves and peripheral nerves
   C. axial and appendicular skeleton
   D. brain and spinal cord

2. Which of the following is **NOT** a component of a neuron?
   A. cell body
   B. synapse
   C. axon
   D. dendrite

3. During the resting state, the inside of the neuron is _____ charged.
   A. negatively
   B. positively
   C. neutral
   D. none of the above

4. During the action potential, the inside of the nerve cell becomes
   A. negative
   B. positive
   C. neutral
   D. none of the above

5. Neurons connect with other neurons at junctions called
   A. neurojunctions
   B. synapses
   C. axons
   D. dendrites

6. The primary neurotransmitters for the autonomic nervous system are
   A. epinephrine
   B. norepinephrine
   C. acetylcholine
   D. B and C

7. The outermost meningeal layer is the
   A. pia mater
   B. arachnoid
   C. subdura
   D. dura mater

Match the six main divisions of the brain with their respective definitions:

8. _____ Cerebrum   **A.** The midbrain

9. _____ Diencephalon   **B.** Contains the higher centers

10. _____ Mesencephalon   **C.** Coordinates motor control and balance

11. _____ Pons   **D.** Contains the thalmus, hypothalmus, limbic system

12. _____ Medulla   **E.** Contains the respiratory and vasomotor centers

13. _____ Cerebellum   **F.** Lies between the midbrain and medulla

14. The right and left hemispheres of the brain are connected by the
   A. medulla oblongata
   B. midbrain
   C. Circle of Willis
   D. corpus callosum

Match the five areas of specialization of the brain with their respective lobe:

15. _____ Temporal   **A.** Personality, motor skills

16. _____ Occipital   **B.** Sensory

17. _____ Frontal   **C.** Speech center

18. _____ Cerebellum   **D.** Coordination and balance

19. _____ Parietal   **E.** Vision

20. The Circle of Willis joins the
   A. carotid and vertebrobasilar circulatory systems
   B. midbrain and brainstem
   C. right and left brain
   D. venous sinuses and jugular veins

21. Nerve fibers that transmit impulses from the brain to the body are called
   A. afferent fibers
   B. efferent fibers
   C. dermatomes
   D. neurotransmitters

22. Each nerve root has a corresponding area of the body to which it supplies sensation. These are called
   A. afferent areas
   B. efferent areas
   C. dermatomes
   D. neurotransmitters

23. The pupils are controlled by which cranial nerve?
   A. First
   B. Third
   C. Fifth
   D. Tenth

24. Which of the following is an early sign of increased intracranial pressure?
   A. Dilated, unreactive pupils
   B. Dilated, reactive pupils
   C. Unilaterally dilated pupil
   D. None of the above

Match the following respiratory patterns with their respective descriptions:

25. _____ Cheyne-Stokes   **A.** Prolonged inspiration

26. _____ Central neurogenic   **B.** No intercostal movement
          hyperventilation

27. _____ Ataxic   **C.** Increase/decrease/apnea

28. _____ Apneustic   **D.** Rapid, deep breathing

29. _____ Diaphragmatic   **E.** Ineffective, muscular coordination

30. Which of the following is true?
   A. Carbon dioxide is a potent vasodilator
   B. Hyperventilation can decrease intracranial pressure
   C. At a $PaCO_2$ of approximately 25 mm/Hg, the cerebral blood vessels constrict
   D. All of the above

31. All of the following are signs of increased intracranial pressure EXCEPT
   A. increased blood pressure
   B. increased pulse rate
   C. decreased respirations
   D. increased temperature

32. A patient who responds to questions, but is disoriented and sluggish is categorized

    A. A
    B. V
    C. P
    D. U

33. Decorticate posturing is characterized by
    A. arms extended, legs extended
    B. arms flexed, legs extended
    C. arms extended, legs flexed
    D. arms flexed, legs flexed

34. A common mnemonic for remembering the causes for coma is
    A. PQRST
    B. AEIOU-TIPS
    C. SLUDGE
    D. ABCDE

35. Inadequate thiamine intake may result in all of the following EXCEPT
    A. Wernicke's syndrome
    B. Kernig's sign
    C. Korsakoff's psychosis
    D. encephalopathy

SCENARIO Your patient is a 56-year-old homeless man who, per bystanders, suffered a seizure. He presents to you on the street, comatose, smelling of alcohol and urine, with vomit and blood around his mouth. Further examination finds him responsive to deep pain with purposeful movement, breathing at 20/minute, heart rate 90 and regular, BP 140/70, pupils equal but sluggish to react. As you prepare to examine him further he seizes once again, full grand mal.

36. The most common cause of seizures is
    A. hypoglycemia
    B. hypoxia
    C. drug overdose
    D. epilepsy

Match the following types of seizures with their respective descriptions:

37. _____ Grand mal   **A.** Brief loss of consciousness

38. _____ Petit mal   **B.** Dysfunction to one area of body

39. _____ Focal motor   **C.** Tonic/clonic extremity movement

40. _____ Psychomotor   **D.** Involves temporal lobe with aura

41. _____ Hysterical   **E.** Can be interrupted, no post-ictal period

42. Status epilepticus is defined as
    A. a seizure due to epilepsy

    B. a seizure that does not stop following diazepam therapy

    C. two or more seizures without a lucid interval

    D. all of the above

43. Which of the above is **NOT RECOMMENDED** in the management of this patient?

    A. IV D₅W

    B. Blood glucose determination

    C. Diazepam IV push

    D. 100% oxygen administration

SCENARIO Your patient is a 75-year-old female who presents at home slumped to one side of the couch. She appears awake, but disoriented. Per her family, she has a long history of hypertension and one stroke. Her respiratory rate is 18, pulse is 90 and regular, BP 170/90, pupils equal and reactive. Her left side is obviously weakened, she slurrs her speech, and has facial drooping. According to her family, these signs are all new.

44. Strokes are caused by

    A. hemorrhage of cerebral blood vessels

    B. thrombus formation

    C. embolism

    D. all of the above

45. Transient ischemic attacks are defined as

    A. minor strokes

    B. temporary strokes

    C. strokes caused by hypoxia

    D. none of the above

46. Patients with strokes commonly present with

    A. bilateral paralysis or paresthesia

    B. polyuria, polydipsia, polyphagia

    C. hemiparesis or hemiplegia

    D. all of the above

47. Hemiplegia means

    A. weakness to the legs

    B. inability to speak

    C. unilateral paralysis

    D. numbness

48. Management of this patient should include

    A. Blood glucose determination

    B. 100% oxygen administration

    C. Cardiac monitoring

    D. all of the above

DRUG DOSE REVIEW

Drug	Adult	Pediatric
50% Dextrose		
Glucagon		
Thiamine		
Diazepam		
Naloxone		
Dexamethasone		

ANSWERS   **1. ANS—D**   *PEC—740*

The central nervous system consists of the brain and spinal cord.

2. ANS—B   *PEC—741*

The fundamental unit of the nervous system is the nerve cell, or neuron. The neuron consists of the cell body containing the nucleus, the dendrites which carry nervous impulses to the cell body, and the axons which transmit nervous impulses away from the cell body.

3. ANS—A   *PEC—741*

The transmission of nervous impulses in the nervous system resembles the conduction of electrical impulses through the heart. In its resting state, the neuron is positively charged on the outside and negatively charged on the inside.

4. ANS—B   *PEC—741*

When stimulated, sodium rapidly enters the cell and potassium rapidly leaves it, producing a positive charge at the entry site.

5. ANS—B   *PEC—741*

The neuron joins with other neurons at junctions called synapses. The neurons do not come into contact with each other at these synapses. Upon reaching the synapse the axon releases a chemical neurotransmitter which crosses the synapse and stimulates the connecting nerve.

6. ANS—D   *PEC—742*

The primary neurotransmitter for the sympathetic nervous system is norepinephrine. The transmitter for the parasympathetic nervous system is acetylcholine.

7. ANS—D   *PEC—744*

The outermost layer of the meninges is the dura mater. An easy way to recall the meningeal layers is to remember that they provide a PAD for the brain (Pia—Arachnoid—Dura)

8. Cerebrum   **B.** Contains the higher centers   *PEC—744*

9. Diencephalon   **D.** Contains the thalmus, hypothalmus, limbic system

10. Mesencephalon   **A.** The midbrain

11. Pons   **F.** Lies between the midbrain and medulla

12. Medulla   **E.** Contains the respiratory and vasomotor centers

13. Cerebellum   **C.** Coordinates motor control and balance

14. ANS—D   *PEC—744*

The right and left hemispheres of the cerebrum are connected by the corpus collosum.

15. Temporal   **C.** Speech center   *PEC—746*

16. Occipital   **E.** Vision

17. Frontal   **A.** Personality, motor skills

18. Cerebellum   **D.** Coordination and balance

19. Parietal   **B.** Sensory

20. ANS—A   *PEC—746*

Blood flow to the brain is provided by two systems. The carotid system is anterior while the vertebrobasilar system is posterior. Both join at the Circle of Willis before entering the substance of the brain.

21. ANS—B   *PEC—746*

Nerve fibers that transmit impulses from the brain to the body are called efferent fibers.

22. ANS—C   *PEC—747*

Each nerve route has a corresponding area of the body called the dermatone to which it supplies sensation.

23. ANS—B   *PEC—750*

The pupils are controlled by the third cranial nerve also called the occulomotor nerve. This nerve follows a long course through the skull and is easily compressed by brain swelling. Thus, it can be an early indicator of increasing intracranial pressure.

24. ANS—C   *PEC—750*

A unilaterally dilated pupil that remains reactive to light may be the earliest sign of increasing intracranial pressure. The patient who presents with or develops the unilaterally dilated pupil is in the immediate transport category.

25. Cheyne-Stokes   **C.** Increase/decrease/apnea   *PEC—750*

26. Central neurogenic   **D.** Rapid, deep breathing
        hyperventilation

27. Ataxic   **E.** Ineffective, muscular coordination

28. Apneustic   **A.** Prolonged inspiration

29. Diaphragmatic   **B.** No intercostal movement

Figure 23-1

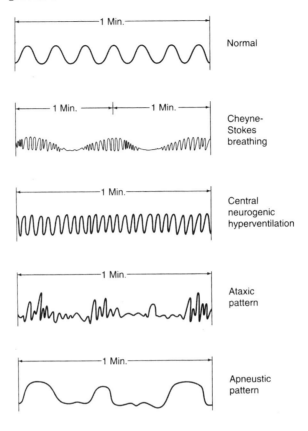

Source: PEC, Figure 23-9.

30. ANS—D   *PEC—751*

The blood level of carbon dioxide has a critical effect on cerebral blood vessels. The normal blood $PaCO_2$ is 40 mm/Hg. Increasing the $PaCO_2$ causes cerebral vasodilatation while decreasing it results in cerebral vasoconstriction. If the patient is poorly ventilated, the $PaCO_2$ will increase causing even further vasodilatation with a subsequent increase in intracranial pressure. Hyperventilation can decrease the $PaCO_2$ to nearly 25 mm/Hg effectively causing vasoconstriction of the cerebral vessels. This will help minimize brain swelling. Therefore, hyperventilate any patient suspected of having increased intracranial pressure at a rate of 24 breaths per minute or greater.

31. ANS—B   *PEC—752*

A person suffering from increased intracranial pressure may exhibit increased blood pressure, decreased pulse, decreased respirations, and an increased temperature.

Comparison of Vital Signs in Shock and Increased ICP		
Vital Signs	**Shock**	**Increased ICP**
Blood Pressure	Decreased	Increased
Pulse	Increased	Decreased
Respirations	Increased	Decreased
LOC	Decreased	Decreased

32. ANS—B   *PEC—753*

A patient who responds to questions but is disoriented and sluggish is categorized V.

33. ANS—B   *PEC—753*

Decorticate posturing is characterized by flexion of the arms and extension of the legs. Decerebrate posturing is characterized by arm and leg extension. Both signify deep cerebral or brainstem injury.

34. ANS—B   *PEC—755*

Unconsciousness or coma is a state in which the patient cannot be aroused even by powerful external stimuli. There generally are only two mechanisms capable of producing alterations in mental status. One, structural lesions and two, toxic-metabolic states. Within these two general categories there are many causes of altered mental status. The mnemonic AEIOUTIPS is an easy way to remember some of them.

A—acidosis alcohol
E—epilepsy
I—infection
O—overdose
U—uremia
T—trauma or tumor
I—insulin
P—psychosis
S—stroke

35. ANS—B   *PEC—758*

Thiamine deficiency may cause Wernicke's syndrome (an acute and reversible encephalopathy) or Korsakoff's Psychosis.

36. ANS—D   *PEC—760*

A seizure is a temporary alteration in behavior due to massive electrical discharge of one or more groups of neurons in the brain. The most common cause is due to idiopathic epilepsy.

37. _____ Grand mal   **C.** Tonic / clonic extremity movement   *PEC—760*

38. _____ Petit mal   **A.** Brief loss of consciousness

39. _____ Focal motor   **B.** Dysfunction to one area of body

40. _____ Psychomotor   **D.** Involves temporal lobe with aura

41. _____ Hysterical   **E.** Can be interrupted, no post-ictal period

42. ANS—C   *PEC—763*

Status epilepticus is a series of two or more generalized motor seizures without an intervening return of consciousness. The most common cause in adults is failure to take prescribed anti-convulsive medications.

43. ANS—A   *PEC—763*

Managing the patient in status epilepticus includes aggressive airway management, oxygenation, IV access with normal saline or Lactated Ringer's, determining blood glucose level and administering 50% dextrose if the patient is hypoglycemic, and administering diazepam IV push.

44. ANS—D   *PEC—763*

A stroke or CVA is a term that describes injury or death of brain tissue, usually due to interruption of cerebral blood flow from either ischemic or hemorrhagic lesions. This may be caused by hemorrhage into the brain tissue, an embolus in the cerebral blood vessels, or thrombus formation that includes arterial supply to the brain.

45. ANS—B   *PEC—765*

Transient ischemic attacks or TIA's are temporary strokes. These are usually caused by emboli which temporarily interfere with the blood supply to the brain producing symptoms of neurologic deficit. These symptoms may last for only a few minutes or for several hours.

46. ANS—C   *PEC—765*

Patients with strokes commonly present with hemiplegia or hemiparesis, unilateral facial droop, speech disturbances, confusion and agitation, eating disturbances, uncoordinated fine motor movements, vision problems, inappropriate behavior with excessive laughing or crying, or coma.

47. ANS—C   *PEC—765*

Hemiplegia means paralysis of one side of the body.

48. ANS—D   *PEC—766*

Management of a patient with stroke symptoms should include determining blood glucose and administering 50% dextrose if the patient is hypoglycemic, administering 100% oxygen, and cardiac monitoring.

DRUG DOSE REVIEW

Drug	Adult	Pediatric
50% Dextrose	25 gm IV	0.5-1 gm/kg IV
Glucagon	0.5-1 mg/kg IM	0.1 mg/kg IM
Thiamine	100 mg IV	rarely used
Diazepam	5-10 mg IV	0.5-2 mg IV
Naloxone	1-2 mg IV	0.01 mg/kg IV
Dexamethasone	4-24 mg IV	1 mg/kg IV

CHAPTER 24

The Acute Abdomen

QUESTIONS

1. The spleen, stomach, and tail of the pancreas are located in the
   A. right upper quadrant
   B. left upper quadrant
   C. right lower quadrant
   D. left lower quadrant

2. The liver, gallbladder, and head of the pancreas are located in the
   A. right upper quadrant
   B. left upper quadrant
   C. right lower quadrant
   D. left lower quadrant

3. The appendix, ascending colon, and small intestine are located in the
   A. right upper quadrant
   B. left upper quadrant
   C. right lower quadrant
   D. left lower quadrant

4. The small intestine and descending colon are located in the
   A. right upper quadrant
   B. left upper quadrant
   C. right lower quadrant
   D. left lower quadrant

5. The abdominal cavity is lined with a membrane called the
   A. perineum
   B. epigastrium
   C. pleura
   D. peritoneum

6. The kidneys are located in the
   A. peritoneum
   B. retroperitoneum
   C. flanks
   D. epigastrium

7. Examples of solid organs are the
   A. stomach and intestines
   B. gallbladder and urinary bladder
   C. uterus and fallopian tubes
   D. liver and spleen

8. The first organ of digestion is the
   A. esophagus
   B. mouth
   C. stomach
   D. small intestine

9. Food moves through the digestive tract in a process called
   A. peristalsis
   B. portal movement
   C. peritonitis
   D. none of the above

Match the components of the digestive system with their respective descriptions:

10. _____ Salivary glands   **A.** Secretes digestive enzymes, insulin, glucagon

11. _____ Liver   **B.** Has no physiological function

12. _____ Gallbladder   **C.** Produce food lubricant and amylase

13. _____ Pancreas   **D.** Stores and excretes bile into the duodenum

14. _____ Appendix   **E.** Stores glycogen, detoxifies many substances

15. The portal system
   A. facilitates food transport through the intestines
   B. transports blood to and from the liver for processing
   C. delivers bile to the intestines for digestion
   D. produces saliva to initiate digestion

Match the components of the genitourinary system with their respective descriptions:

16. _____ Kidney   **A.** Stores urine

17. _____ Ureter   **B.** Filters blood and produces urine

18. _____ Urinary bladder   **C.** Connects bladder to outside

19. _____ Urethra   **D.** Connects kidney with bladder

Match the components of the female reproductive system with their respective descriptions:

20. _____ Ovaries   **A.** Site of implantation and development of the fetus

21. _____ Fallopian tubes **B.** External female genitalia

22. _____ Uterus   **C.** Produces the ovum and female hormones

23. _____ Vagina   **D.** Connect the ovaries to the uterus

24. _____ Vulva   **E.** Birth canal, organ for copulation

Match the components of the male reproductive system with their respective descriptions:

25. _____ Testes   **A.** Sperm reservoir

26. _____ Epididymis   **B.** Transports sperm from testes to urethra

27. _____ Prostate   **C.** Male organ for copulation

28. _____ Vas deferens   **D.** Produce male hormones and sperm

29. _____ Urethra   **E.** Produces fluid to transport sperm

30. _____ Penis   **F.** Connects uninary bladder to the outside

31. Urine flow may be obstructed in the male by the presence of
   A. epididymis
   B. prostatitis
   C. testitis
   D. testicular torsion

32. Your patient, an alcoholic with a long history of liver damage, presents with painless bright red upper GI bleeding. The most likely cause of the bleeding is
   A. gastritis
   B. peptic ulcer disease
   C. esophageal varices
   D. diverticulosis

33. This condition results from
   A. fatty foods
   B. congenital problems
   C. calcium deposits
   D. portal hypertension

34. Your patient presents with epigastric pain, belching, and indigestion which improves after eating. This condition, caused by inflammation of the stomach lining, and associated with alcohol ingestion, stress, or drug abuse is known as
   A. diverticulitis
   B. pancreatitis
   C. gastritis
   D. pylonephritis

35. Treatment of this condition may include
   A. avoidance of alcohol
   B. histamine 2 blockers
   C. cimetidine
   D. all of the above

36. Your patient presents with severe lower right abdominal pain, anorexia, nausea, vomiting, fever, and rebound tenderness may be suffering from
   A. gastritis
   B. appendicitis
   C. cholecystitis
   D. pylonephritis

37. Epigastric pain condition characterized by inflammation of the gall-bladder is known as
   A. pylonephritis
   B. cholecystitis
   C. gastritis
   D. hepatitis

38. Coffee ground emesis is indicative of
   A. lower GI bleeding
   B. upper GI bleeding
   C. bowel obstruction
   D. diverticulosis

39. Bright red bleeding into the stool is indicative of
   A. lower GI bleeding
   B. upper GI bleeding
   C. bowel obstruction
   D. esophageal varices

40. Your patient with dull right upper quadrant pain (unrelated to eating), malaise, clay-colored stools, and jaundice may be suffering from
   A. cholecystitis
   B. hepatitis
   C. pancreatitis
   D. diverticulitis

41. Your patient with diffuse abdominal pain and back pain, with a pulsating mass noted to the left of midline may be suffering from
   A. diverticulosis
   B. diverticulitis
   C. bowel obstruction
   D. aortic aneurysm

42. Women are more prone to bladder infections than men because
   A. their urethra are shorter
   B. their urethra are longer
   C. their ureters are shorter
   D. their ureters are longer

43. A kidney infection is known as
   A. diverticulitis
   B. hepatitis
   C. pylonephritis
   D. epididymitis

44. Which of the following is a complication of chronic renal failure?
   A. Fluid volume overload
   B. Hypokalemia
   C. Polyuria
   D. All of the above

45. Your patient in chronic renal failure may present with
   A. ascites
   B. rales in the lung bases
   C. jugular venous distension
   D. all of the above

46. Uremia is a condition manifested by
   A. blood in the urine
   B. uric acid in the blood
   C. fluid in the abdominal cavity
   D. calculi in the urine

47. Your female patient who complains of lower abdominal pain while walking and during sexual intercourse, fever, and vaginal discharge may be suffering from
   A. ovarian cyst
   B. mittelschmerz
   C. epididymitis
   D. pelvic inflammatory disease

48. The abdominal pain associated with the release of the egg from the ovary is known as
   A. epididymitis
   B. mittelschmerz
   C. prostatitis
   D. cystitis

49. Rebound tenderness is indicative of
   A. peritoneal irritation
   B. aortic aneurysm
   C. bowel obstruction
   D. ectopic pregnancy

50. Your patient's blood pressure is 120/80 and pulse is 80 lying down. When you sit him up his blood pressure drops to 100/60 and his pulse rises to 100. This is known as a
   A. hypotensive disorder
   B. positive tilt test
   C. normal phenomenon
   D. rebound mechanism

51. The P in the mnemonic PQRST refers to
A. pain
B. pallor
C. provocative
D. pulse

52. The process of hemodialysis is based on the principle of
A. diffusion
B. osmosis
C. homeostasis
D. all of the above

53. Possible complications from hemodialysis include
A. disequilibrium syndrome
B. hypotension
C. air embolism
D. all of the above

ANSWERS

1. ANS—B *PEC—771*

The spleen, stomach, and pancreas are located in the left upper quadrant.

2. ANS—A *PEC—771*

The liver, gallbladder, and head of the pancreas are located in the right upper quadrant.

3. ANS—C *PEC—771*

The appendix, ascending colon, and small intestine are located in the right lower quadrant.

4. ANS—D *PEC—771*

The small intestine and descending colon are located in the left lower quadrant.

5. ANS—D *PEC—771*

The abdominal cavity is lined with a membrane called the peritoneum. Most organs are located within this membrane.

6. ANS—B *PEC—771*

The kidneys are located in the space behind the peritoneum, called the retroperitoneum.

7. ANS—D *PEC—772*

Examples of solid organs are the liver, spleen, pancreas, kidneys, adrenals, and ovaries in the female.

8. ANS—B *PEC—772*

The first organ of digestion is the mouth. It breaks down food into smaller particles, secretes saliva for lubrication, and amylase for digestion.

9. ANS—A *PEC—773*

Food moves through the intestines through a process called peristalsis.

10. Salivary glands   **C.** Produce food lubricant and amylase *PEC—773*

11. Liver

E. Stores glycogen, detoxifies many substances

12. Gallbladder

D. Stores and excretes bile into the duodenum

13. Pancreas

A. Secretes digestive enzymes, insulin, glucagon

14. Appendix

B. Has no physiological function

15. ANS—B   *PEC—773*

The portal system is a specialized circulatory system within the abdomen. This system drains blood from parts of the intestines and transports it to the liver where it is filtered and processed.

16. Kidney

B. Filters blood and produces urine   *PEC—774*

17. Ureter

D. Connects kidney with bladder

18. Urinary bladder

A. Stores urine

19. Urethra

C. Connects bladder to outside

20. Ovaries

C. Produces the ovum and female   *PEC—775*
hormones

21. Fallopian tubes

D. Connect the ovaries to the uterus

22. Uterus

A. Site of implantation and development of the fetus

23. Vagina

E. Birth canal, organ for copulation

24. Vulva

B. External female genitalia

25. Testes

D. Produce male hormones and sperm *PEC—776*

26. Epididymis

A. Sperm reservoir

27. Prostate

E. Produces fluid to transport sperm

28. Vas deferens

B. Transports sperm from testes to urethra

29. Urethra

F. Connects urinary bladder to the outside

30. Penis

C. Male organ for copulation

31. ANS—B   *PEC—776*

Urine flow may be obstructed in the male by the presence of prostatitis. The prostrate is a small gland at the base of the bladder responsible for production of fluid to transport sperm. In older men it can become enlarged and, at certain times, obstruct urine flow.

32. ANS—C   *PEC—776*

Esophageal varices are swollen veins in the lower third of the esophagus. They result from increased pressure in the portal circulation. Diseases of the liver such as alcoholic cirrhosis can slow portal circulation causing engorgement of the veins in the lower esophagus and the rectum. The most common presentation is painless, bright red, upper gastrointestinal bleeding.

33. ANS—D   *PEC—776*

Esophageal varices results from increased back pressure in the hepatic arteries and veins.

34. ANS—C   *PEC—776*

Gastritis is an inflammation of the lining of the stomach. It results from increased gastric acid secretion and is associated with alcohol ingestion, drugs, and other factors. The patient will often complain of epigastric pain, belching, and indigestion. The pain often improves after eating.

35. ANS—D   *PEC—776*

Treatment of gastritis may include avoidance of alcohol, administration of antacids, and histamine blocking drugs such as cimetidine (Tagamet).

36. ANS—B   *PEC—776*

Appendicitis is the inflammation of the appendix. The patient suffering appendicitis will usually complain of right lower quadrant abdominal pain, nausea, vomiting, fever, and anorexia. The peritoneum will generally become inflamed and rebound tenderness will be present.

37. ANS—B   *PEC—779*

Inflammation of the gallbladder is called cholecystitis. It usually occurs when gall stones lodge in the cystic duct that drains the gallbladder.

38. ANS—B   *PEC—778*

Coffee ground emesis is indicative of upper GI bleeding. The blood turns dark brown as it mixes with hydrochloric acid in the stomach.

39. ANS—A   *PEC—778*

Bright red bleeding into the stool is indicative of lower GI bleeding. Causes of lower GI bleeding include tumors, bleeding from diverticula in the colon, hemorrhoids, and rectal fissures.

40. ANS—B   *PEC—779*

Hepatitis is an inflammation or infection of the liver. The patient will often complain of dull, right upper quadrant abdominal tenderness usually unrelated to digestion to food with malaise, decreased appetite, clay-colored stools, and jaundice.

41. ANS—D   *PEC—779*

Weakness in the wall of the descending aorta can occur with age and result in a ballooning of the wall of the vessel. This ballooning may increase in size and eventually rupture. The patient with an abdominal aortic aneurysm is usually with an older person who complains of diffusive abdominal pain and severe back pain. A pulsating abdominal mass may also be noted.

42. ANS—A   *PEC—780*

Urinary tract infections occur frequently. The UTI occurs more often in females because of the relatively short urethra compared to that in the males.

43. ANS—C   *PEC—780*

Pylonephritis is an infection of the kidney.

44. ANS—A   *PEC—781*

Complications of chronic renal failure include fluid overload, hyperkalemia, uremic pericarditis, pericardial tamponade, and uremic encephalopathy.

45. ANS—D   *PEC—781*

The patient in chronic renal failure may present with severe dyspnea, neck vein distention, ascites, and rales at the lung bases.

46. ANS—B   *PEC—781*

Uremia is a condition characterized by increased uric acid in the blood. This is a common complication from chronic renal failure.

47. ANS—D   *PEC—781*

Pelvic inflammatory disease is an infection of the female reproductive organs. It is usually sexually transmitted. The patient presents with fever, chills, lower abdominal pain, and vaginal bleeding or discharge. In addition, the patient may complain of pain on walking or pain with intercourse.

48. ANS—B   *PEC—782*

Mittelschmerz is abdominal pain that is associated with release of the egg from the ovary. It occurs halfway through the menstrual cycle.

49. ANS—A   *PEC—784*

Any patient complaining of an acute abdomen should be checked for rebound tenderness. This can be done by slowly palpating each abdominal quadrant, then quickly withdraw your hand allowing the abdominal wall to return to its normal position. If this causes pain, the patient has rebound tenderness, usually suggestive of peritoneal irritation.

50. ANS—B   *PEC—785*

The patient with an acute abdomen should also be given a tilt test. First take the patient's blood pressure and pulse in the supine position. Then repeat both with the patient in the seated position. A positive tilt test is an increase in the pulse rate of 15 beats per minute or a drop in the systolic blood pressure of 15 mm Hg when the patient is moved from the supine to the sitting position. A positive tilt test indicates relative hypovolemia.

51. ANS—C   *PEC—786*

The P refers to provocative factors: what initiates or aggravates the pain, makes it worse, or makes it better.

52. ANS—D   *PEC—787*

The process of hemodialysis is based on the principles of diffusion, osmosis, and homeostasis.

53. ANS—D   *PEC—788*

Possible complications from hemodialysis include hypotension caused by dehydration, sepsis or blood loss, chest pain or dysrhythmias, caused by potassium intoxication, disequilibrium syndrome, and air embolism which may occur when negative pressure develops in the venous side of the dialysis tubing.

CHAPTER 25

Anaphylaxis

QUESTIONS

1. Anaphylaxis is defined as
  A. an acute, generalized, violent reaction
  B. an antigen/antibody process
  C. a life-threatening emergency
  D. all of the above

2. Any substance capable of producing an immune system response is a/an
  A. antibody
  B. antigen
  C. receptor
  D. idiosyncrasy

3. The antibody responsible for producing allergic and anaphylactic response is the
  A. IgA
  B. IgE
  C. IgM
  D. IgG

4. The antibody that has "memory" and recognizes repeat invasions of foreign substances are the
  A. IgA
  B. IgE
  C. IgM
  D. IgG

5. Which of the following is true regarding vaccines?
  A. They stimulate antibody production
  B. They are an inactivated version of the original infection
  C. Some last a lifetime
  D. All of the above

6. Histamine receptors are located in the
  A. airways
  B. peripheral blood vessels
  C. digestive tract
  D. all of the above

7. Histamine causes all of the following physiological reactions EXCEPT
  A. bronchodilation
  B. increased peristalsis
  C. capillary leaking
  D. vasodilation

8. The person with anaphylaxis may exhibit all of the following signs and symptoms EXCEPT
  A. hypertension
  B. stridor
  C. urticaria
  D. abdominal cramping

9. Angioedema is best described as
  A. facial swelling
  B. third cranial nerve paralysis
  C. generalized body hives
  D. excema of the neck

10. The anaphylactic shock patient should be managed with
  A. aggressive airway management
  B. epinephrine and diphenhydramine
  C. oxygen 100%
  D. all of the above

11. Epinephrine causes all of the following EXCEPT
  A. bronchodilation
  B. peripheral blood vessel constriction
  C. heart rate decrease
  D. contractile force increase

12. Diphenhydramine is given in anaphylaxis because it
  A. blocks histamine receptor sites
  B. enhances the effects of epinephrine
  C. renders the antigen inactive
  D. produces permanent immunity

13. In addition to epinephrine and diphenhydramine the medical control physician may order corticosteroids because they
  A. slow histamine release
  B. reduce capillary leakage
  C. reduce edema and swelling
  D. all of the above

14. Which of the following best describes the use of PASG in anaphylaxis?
  A. It should be used with caution
  B. It may exacerbate pulmonary edema
  C. It will increase peripheral vascular resistance
  D. All of the above

DRUG DOSE REVIEW

Drug	Adult	Pediatric
Epinephrine 1:1000		
Epinephrine 1:10000		
Diphenhydramine		
Methylprednisolone		

ANSWERS

1. ANS—D *PEC—794*

Anaphylaxis is an acute, generalized, violent antigen-antibody reaction that may be rapidly fatal even with prompt and appropriate emergency care.

2. ANS—B *PEC—795*

An antigen is any substance capable of producing an immune response. Examples include bacteria, viruses, drug molecules, animal secretions or serum, blood, and many others.

3. ANS—B *PEC—795*

The IgE (immunoglobulin G) antibody contributes to allergic and anaphylactic responses.

4. ANS—D *PEC—795*

The IgG (immunoglobulin G) antibody has "memory" and recognizes repeat invasions of the antigen.

5. ANS—D *PEC—795*

A vaccine is an agent that when injected will produce an immune response. Most vaccines are inactivated forms of the original virus or bacteria. Some vacines, such as chicken pox, last a lifetime. Others, such as tetanus, must be repeated via boosters.

6. ANS—D *PEC—797*

Histamine 1 receptors are located in the lower airways and peripheral blood vessels. Histamine 2 receptors are located in the stomach.

7. ANS—A *PEC—797*

Histamine causes bronchoconstriction, capillary leaking from increased permeability, peripheral vasodilation, increased gastric secretion, and increased movement of food through the digestive tract.

8. ANS—A *PEC—797*

Hypertension does not occur in true anaphylaxis. One of the cardinal effects is massive vasodilation which results in hypotension.

9. ANS—A   *PEC—798*

Peripheral vasodilation and increased capillary permeability cause swelling in the face and mucous membranes. This is called angioedema.

10. ANS—D   *PEC—800*

The patient in anaphylactic shock should receive aggressive airway management, 100% oxygenation, epinephrine SC or IV, diphenhydramine IV, and PASG as needed.

11. ANS—C   *PEC—800*

Epinephrine is the drug of choice for anaphylaxis because it reverses the effects of histamine by causing bronchodilation and peripheral vasoconstriction. It will also increase heart rate and strength of contractions.

12. ANS—A   *PEC—801*

Diphenhydramine is given in anaphylaxis because it competes with histamine at the receptor sites. By blocking the effects of histamine, you stop the life-threatening allergic response.

13. ANS—D   *PEC—802*

Corticosteroids, such as methylprednisolone, hydrocortisone, and dexamethasone play a role in stopping the inflammation response. They slow histamine release from the mast cells, slow capillary leaking, thus reducing tissue edema. Since steroids do not have an immediate effect, they are not considered a first-line medication.

14. ANS—D   *PEC—802*

The use of the PASG in anaphylaxis is controversial. While it will increase peripheral vasacular restsiance, it may also worsen pulmonary edema.

DRUG DOSE REVIEW

Drug	Adult	Pediatric
Epinephrine 1:1000	0.3–0.5 mg SC	0.01 mg/kg SC
Epinephrine 1:10000	0.3–0.5 mg IV	0.01 mg/kg IV
Diphenhydramine	25–50 mg IV/IM	2–5 mg/kg IV/IM
Methylprednisolone	125–250 mg IV	30 mg/kg IV

CHAPTER 26

Toxicology and Substance Abuse

QUESTIONS

1. The most common route of entry for toxic exposure is
A. inhalation
B. ingestion
C. surface absorption
D. injection

2. Toxic gases such as methyl chloride, chlorine, and carbon monoxide enter the bloodstream through the
A. blood brain barrier
B. skin
C. alveolar-capillary membrane
D. intestinal tract

3. Hymenoptera deliver their poisonous substances through the
A. blood brain barrier
B. skin
C. alveolar-capillary membrane
D. intestinal tract

4. Which of the following is an advantage of having a poison control center?
A. It is staffed by poison control specialists
B. It is available 24 hours a day
C. It offers the most current information
D. All of the above

5. The poison antidote that works by absorbing large amounts of poisonous molecules in the stomach is
   A. syrup of ipecac
   B. naloxone
   C. activated charcoal
   D. amyl nitrate

6. An agent that causes emesis is
   A. syrup of ipecac
   B. naloxone
   C. activated charcoal
   D. amyl nitrate

7. In which of the following circumstances should you induce vomiting?
   A. Patients who have ingested strong acids or alkalis
   B. Patients with a decreased level of consciousness
   C. Pregnant patients
   D. Patients who have ingested aspirin and acetaminophen

8. The "coma cocktail" consists of
   A. 5% dextrose and 0.45% NS
   B. Naloxone, thiamine, 50% dextrose
   C. 50% dextrose and diazepam
   D. Naloxone, thiamine, Narcan

9. Patients exhibiting extrapyramidal effects from taking phenothiazines should receive
   A. diazepam
   B. a "coma cocktail"
   C. syrup of ipecac
   D. diphenhydramine

10. A lethal type of food poisoning caused by improper food storage methods is
   A. clostridium botulinum
   B. salmonella
   C. E coli
   D. scomboid

11. Which of the following describes the pathophysiology of cyanide poisoning?
   A. Cyanide binds with hemoglobin, preventing oxygen transport
   B. Cyanide paralyzes the central nervous system
   C. Cyanide prevents cellular use of oxygen
   D. Cyanide can only be inhaled

12. A cyanide antidote kit should contain
   A. amyl nitrate ampules
   B. sodium nitrite solution
   C. a sodium thiosulfate solution
   D. all of the above

13. Freon gas primarily affects the
   A. central nervous system

    B. respiratory system

    C. heart

    D. digestive system

14. Hymenoptera is a class of insects that includes all of the following **EXCEPT**

    A. spiders

    B. ants

    C. bees

    D. wasps

SCENARIO Your patient is a 63-year-old homeless male who is an habitual ambulance customer. This evening you find him slumped against a tree in the park, seemingly unconscious. He is alive, but responds neither to voice or deep pain. Next to him you find a jar labeled "wood alcohol." His BP is 150/90, pulse 90, respirations 40. He lies in a pool of vomit and reeks of alcohol.

15. This patient is most likely suffering from

    A. alcohol intoxication

    B. acute methanol poisoning

    C. cyanide poisnoning

    D. none of the above

16. Treatment for this patient may include all of the following **EXCEPT**

    A. contacting poison control

    B. 30-60 ml of 86 proof whiskey

    C. 50 mEq sodium bicarbonate

    D. 100 mg thiamine

SCENARIO Yourt patient is a 26-year-old male who was barbecueing in his garage with the overhead door half closed. His wife called 911 because he began acting strangely and vomited. You find him walking around the house, disoriented, complaining of a severe headache and nausea.

17. This man is most likely suffering from

    A. carbon monoxide poisoning

    B. acute methanol intoxication

    C. cyanide poisoning

    D. organophosphate poisoning

18. Management of this patient includes

    A. removal from the toxic environment

    B. oxygen administration

    C. transport to a hyperbaric chamber

    D. all of the above

SCENARIO Your patient is a 25-year-old rock climber who was bitten by a rattlesnake and walked to call for help (1 mile). She presents on the ground complaining of weakness, dizzyness, and pain at the injection site. She has fang marks on her left leg with oozing. She is nauseated and has vomited twice. Her BP is 80/50, pulse is 120 and weak, skin cool, pale, and clammy to the touch.

19. Rattlesnakes are members of what class of snakes?
  A. Hymenoptera
  B. Pit vipers
  C. Elapidae
  D. Coral

20. Which of the following statements is true regarding rattlesnakes?
  A. Their bite can result in death within 30 minutes
  B. Their bites seldom cause systemic reactions
  C. All rattlesnakes have rattles
  D. All rattlesnake bites inject poisonous venom

21. Management of a rattlesnake bite includes all of the following EXCEPT
  A. application of a constricting band proximal to the wound
  B. keeping the patient calm
  C. application of ice, compression, and elevation to the wound
  D. immobilizing the extremity

SCENARIO Your patient is a 49-year-old female who was working in her garden trying to apply an insect killer to her roses. She was not wearing gloves and got much of the insecticide on her skin. She presents on the ground, disoriented, with vomit and drool on her shirt. She is incontinent of urine. Her BP is 100/60, pulse rate is 55, respirations are 20, skin is pale and wet, pupils constricted.

22. This patient should be suspected of having
  A. cyanide poisoning
  B. organophosphate poisoning
  C. snake bite reaction
  D. bee sting reaction

23. The best explanation for her vital signs is a/an
  A. sympathetic nervous system response
  B. parasympathetic nervous system response
  C. compensatory shock mechanism
  D. antigen/antibody response

24. Treatment for this patient should include all of the following EXCEPT
  A. inducing vomiting
  B. vigorous airway suctioning
  C. atropine IV
  D. contacting poison control

SCENARIO Your patient is a 35-year-old confirmed alcoholic who calls you 2 days after leaving the detox unit. He presents with general weakness, tremors of the hands, sweating, and very anxious. He complains of nausea and vomiting and that he cannot sleep. His skin is cool and clammy, BP—140/70, pulse 90, respirations 20. He claims he sees pink elephants behind you and generally acts very strangely.

25. This patient is most likely suffering from
   A. acute psychosis
   B. delusions
   C. acute alcohol withdrawal
   D. ethylene glycol poisoning

DRUG DOSE REVIEW

Drug	Adult	Pediatric
Ipecac		
Activated Charcoal		

ANSWERS

1. ANS—B   *PEC—807*

Ingestion is the most common route of entry for toxic exposure. Frequently ingested poisons include household products, petroleum-based agents (gasoline and paint), cleaning agents (alkalies and soaps), cosmetics, prescribed drugs, plants, and foods.

2. ANS—C   *PEC—808*

Inhalation of a poison results in rapid absorption of the toxic agent through the alveolar-capillary membrane. Commonly inhaled poisons include toxic gases, carbon monoxide, ammonia, chlorine, freon, toxic vapors, fumes, or aerosols, carbon tetrachloride, methyl chloride, tear gas, mustard gas, and nitrous oxide.

3. ANS—B   *PEC—808*

Most poisonings by injection result from the bites and stings of insects and animals. Most insects that sting and bite belong to the class hymenoptera, which includes bees, hornets, yellow jackets, wasps, and ants.

4. ANS—D   *PEC—809*

Poison control centers have been set up across the United States and Canada to assist in the treatment of poison victims and to provide information on new products and new treatment recommendations. Centers are usually staffed by physicians, pharmacists, nurses, or poison control specialists trained in toxicology and are available to callers 24 hours-a-day.

5. ANS—C   *PEC—810*

Activated charcoal promotes gastrointestinal decontamination via its large surface area that can absorb molecules from the offending poison.

6. ANS—A   *PEC—810*

In some cases of ingestion, emetic agents such as syrup of ipecac can be used to empty the stomach. Syrup of ipecac works by irritating the lining of the stomach and by stimulating the vomit center in the medulla.

7. ANS—D   *PEC—812*

If the patient has ingested the toxic substance within three to six hours of your arrival, the poison control center may recommend inducement of vomiting in the field. Vomiting should not be induced for patients who have ingested strong alkalis or acids, patients with a decreased level of consciousness, or those who are pregnant.

8. ANS—B   *PEC—814*

The "coma cocktail" consists of naloxone, thiamine, and 50% dextrose.

9. ANS—D   *PEC—814*

Physicians sometimes prescribe a group of drugs called phenothiazines. These drugs, however, cause allergic reactions in patients that are sensitive to them. These reactions may be alleviated with the administration of diphenhydramine.

10. ANS—A   *PEC—815*

Clostridium botulinum, the world's most toxic poison, occurs in cases of improper food storage methods such as canning.

11. ANS—C   *PEC—818*

Cyanide inflicts its damage by inhibiting cytochrome oxidase, an enzyme vital to cellular use of oxygen. Once cyanide enters the body it acts as a cellular asphyxiant.

12. ANS—D   *PEC—819*

A cyanide antidote kit should contain amyl nitrate ampules, a sodium nitrate, and a sodium thiosulfate solution.

13. ANS—C   *PEC—819*

Freon is a common refrigerant which causes direct cardiac toxicity by the sudden release of endogenous catecholamines. Its effect on the heart is a variety of ventricular ectopic activity including PVCs, ventricular tachycardia, and ventricular fibrillation.

14. ANS—A   *PEC—821*

Hymenoptera is a class of insects that includes wasps, bees, hornets, and ants.

15. ANS—B   *PEC—816*

Methanol is used in a variety of automotive products and cooking fuel that is toxic when ingested. Consumption of as little as 4 cc of methanol has produced blindness while 10 cc has caused death. It is used occasionally by chronic alcoholics trying to get intoxicated.

16. ANS—B   *PEC—816*

Treatment of methanol poisoning includes contacting the poison control center and considering 30-60 milliliters of 86 proof ethanol (vodka, whisky, gin, etc.) and 50mEq of sodium bicarbonate.

17. ANS—A   *PEC—819*

Carbon monoxide is an odorless, tasteless gas that is often the by-product of incomplete combustion. It has more than 200 times the infinity of oxygen to bind with red blood cells hemoglobin producing carboxyhemoglobin. Once this molecule has bound with hemoglobin, it is very resistant to removal and causes hypoxia.

18. ANS—D   *PEC—819*

Management of the carbon monoxide poisoning includes removing the patient from the toxic environment, administering high concentrations of oxygen, and transporting the victim as soon as possible to a hyperbaric chamber.

19. ANS—B   *PEC—825*

Rattlesnakes are members of the pit viper class. Pit vipers are so named because of the instinctive pit between the eye and the nostril on each side of the head.

20. ANS—A   *PEC—826*

A severe bite of a pit viper such as a rattlesnake can result in death from shock within 30 minutes.

21. ANS—C   *PEC—827*

Management of a rattlesnake bite includes applying a constrictive band proximal to the wound on the extremity, keeping the patient calm, and immobilizing the extremity.

22. ANS—B   *PEC—829*

Organophosphates are used as insecticides in residential and commercial agriculture.

23. ANS—B   *PEC—829*

Organophosphates inactivate cholinesterase at the synaptic junction causing elevated levels of the neurotransmitter acetylcholine. This produces a parasympathetic nervous system response.

24. ANS—A   *PEC—830*

Treatment of this patient includes aggressive airway management to include vigorous suctioning, contacting poison control, and administering atropine IV.

25. ANS—C   *PEC—835*

The alcoholic may suffer a withdrawal reaction from either abrupt continuous ingestion after prolonged use or from a rapid fall in the blood alcohol level after acute intoxication. Withdrawal symptoms can occur several hours after sudden abstinence and can last up to 5-7 days.

DRUG DOSE REVIEW

Drug	Adult	Pediatric
Ipecac	30 ml po	< 1 yr—5-10 ml po > 1 yr—15 ml po
Activated Charcoal	50 gm slurry	50 gm slurry

CHAPTER 27

Infectious Diseases

QUESTIONS

1. A small, unicellular organism that causes an infection that is treatable by antibiotics is a
  A. bacteria
  B. virus
  C. fungus
  D. parasite

2. A microscopic agent of infection that invades cells that is not treatable by antibiotics is a
  A. bacteria
  B. virus
  C. fungus
  D. parasite

3. Biological agents such as yeasts and molds are examples of
  A. bacteria
  B. viruses
  C. fungi
  D. parasites

4. A key organ in the lymphatic system that filters red blood cells and helps form antibodies is the
  A. liver
  B. spleen

    C. pancreas

    D. gallbladder

5. Examples of blood-borne diseases include all of the following **EXCEPT**

    A. hepatitis A

    B. hepatitis B

    C. AIDS

    D. syphilis

6. Examples of airborne diseases include all of the following **EXCEPT**

    A. meningitis

    B. tuberculosis

    C. measles

    D. hepatitis A

7. Which of the following is true regarding infectious agents?

    A. Some organisms may remain infectious on a stretcher surface for weeks after contamination

    B. Some agents die soon after exposure to light and air

    C. Paramedics may play a major role in curbing infectious disease transmission

    D. All of the above.

8. In order to test a paramedic for immunity to hepatitis B, it is necessary to

    A. test for the presence of antigens

    B. wait for symptoms to occur

    C. test for the presence of antibodies

    D. none of the above

9. The paramedic should be concerned about infection control procedures

    A. before the incident

    B. during the incident

    C. after the incident

    D. all of the above

10. Appropriate universal precautions include

    A. never recapping needles

    B. wearing gloves during all patient contact

    C. isolating all body fluids

    D. all of the above

11. Your patient who presents with general malaise, low grade fever, headache, and a stiff or sore neck may be suffering from

    A. hepatitis A

    B. meningitis

    C. tuberculosis

    D. AIDS

12. Meningitis is spread primarily by which of the following methods?

    A. A needle stick

    B. Eating contaminated food

    C. Blood transfusion

D. A sneeze or cough

13. A yearly PPD test is necessary to monitor the presence of which disease?
A. Hepatitis B
B. Meningitis
C. Tuberculosis
D. AIDS

14. The childhood disease characterized by fever and salivary gland swelling is
A. mumps
B. rubeola
C. varicella
D. chicken pox

15. Chicken pox, a childhood disease, may manifest itself later in life in a disease called
A. varicella
B. shingles
C. rubeola
D. rubella

16. The type of hepatitis transmitted from restaurant workers who fail to wash their hands before handling food is
A. A
B. B
C. C
D. D

17. The sexually transmitted disease characterized by lower abdominal pain, yellowish vaginal discharge, and pain with intercourse is
A. syphilis
B. gonorrhea
C. AIDS
D. herpes

18. Cold sores are a form of
A. chlamydia
B. gonorrhea
C. herpes
D. syphilis

19. Which of the following statements is true regarding AIDS?
A. It is transmitted via most body fluids
B. Paramedics are included in the high-risk group for contracting this disease
C. The disease weakens the body's immune system by affecting t lymphocytes
D. All of the above

20. The most frequent source of AIDS infection in health care workers is
A. airborne droplets

    B. accidental needlestick
    C. endotracheal intubation
    D. mouth-to-mask ventilation

ANSWERS   **1. ANS—A**   *PEC—841*

Bacteria are small unicellular organisms that live throughout the environment and frequently cause infection. Most bacterial infections respond to treatment with drugs called antibiotics.

2. ANS—B   *PEC—841*

Most infections are caused by biological agents called viruses. Viruses are referred to as intracellular parasites since they must invade the cells of the organism they infect. Once inside a cell they use the various cellular enzymes to replicate and produce more viruses. They cannot produce outside of the host cell, and unlike bacteria, they are very difficult to treat. Once a virus infects a cell, it can only be killed by destroying the infected cell. Drugs have not yet been developed that can selectively destroy cells infected by viruses while simultaneously leaving uninfected cells unharmed.

3. ANS—C   *PEC—842*

Biological agents such as yeasts and molds are examples of fungi. Fungi are biological agents that can cause human infection, usually found on the skin.

4. ANS—B   *PEC—843*

The lympathic system is a separate circulatory system which helps transport materials between the tissues and the blood. Its job is to rid the body of inactivated or dead infectious agents filtered out through the capillaries. The key organ in the lympathic system is the spleen. The solid organ lies in the left upper quadrant of the abdomen. It filters red blood cells and participates in the formation of cells that manufacture antibodies.

5. ANS—A   *PEC—843*

Blood-borne diseases are those transmitted by contact with the blood or body fluids of an infected person. Blood-borne diseases include AIDS, hepatitis B, hepatitis C, hepatitis D, and syphilis.

6. ANS—D   *PEC—843*

Airborne diseases are those transmitted through the air on droplets expelled during a productive cough or sneeze. Examples of airborne diseases include tuberculosis, meningitis, mumps, measles, rubella, and chicken pox.

7. ANS—D   *PEC—844*

Paramedics play a major role in curbing infectious disease transmission. Some organisms may remain infectious on a stretcher surface for weeks after contamination while others die soon after exposures to light and air.

8. ANS—C   *PEC—844*

In order to test a paramedic for immunity to hepatitis B, it is necessary to test for the presence of antibodies.

9. ANS—D   *PEC—845*

There are four phases of infection control in prehospital care. These include preparations before, response to, operations at, and recovery from emergency incidents.

10. ANS—D   *PEC—847*

Appropriate universal precautions include never recapping needles, wearing gloves during all patient contact, and isolating all body fluids.

11. ANS—B   *PEC—850*

Meningitis is the most common central nervous system infection encountered in prehospital care. The disease infects the lining of the brain and spinal cord. It occurs more frequently in children, but adults can also be victims. It's caused by bacteria, viruses, and occasional fungi.

12. ANS—D   *PEC—851*

Meningitis is primarily transmitted through airborne droplets expelled by a productive cough or sneeze.

13. ANS—C   *PEC—851*

A Purified Protein Derivative (PPD) test is necessary to test for tuberculosis. It consists of placing a small amount of protein from the tuberculosis bacteria into the skin. After 48 hours the site is examined. If there's a firm raised area greater than 10 millimeters in diameter, the patient is said to have converted indicating prior exposure to tuberculosis.

14. ANS—A   *PEC—854*

The childhood disease characterized by fever and salivary gland swelling is called mumps. The infection results from the mumps virus which is transmitted usually through the saliva of an infected person.

15.ANS—B   *PEC—854*

Chicken pox, a childhood disease, may manifest itself later in life in a disease called shingles. Once a person has been infected he or she is usually immune for life, but the virus may remain in the body dormant for many years generally living in nerves along the back. In later life, the virus may become active causing illness known as shingles.

16. ANS—A   *PEC—855*

Hepatitis A is the most common form of hepatitis. The route of transmission is usually fecal-oral. Patients usually become infected by eating food contaminated with stool from another person infected with the disease.

17. ANS—B   *PEC—857*

Gonorrhea is a common sexually transmitted disease. It is characterized by burning urination, yellowish vaginal discharge, and pain with walking or movement such as intercourse.

18. ANS—C   *PEC—858*

Cold sores are a form of the herpes simplex type one virus. These sores are usually found around the mouth and lips.

19. ANS—D   *PEC—858*

AIDS is a world-wide epidemic and a virtual threat to every individual on this planet caused by the human immuno-deficiency virus HIV. It is transmitted through most body secretions and by most body fluids. It weakens the body's immune system by affecting the t lymphocytes. Paramedics are included in the high-risk group for contracting this disease.

20. ANS—B *PEC—859*

The most frequent source of AIDS infection of health care workers is the accidental needle stick.

CHAPTER 28

Environmental Emergencies

QUESTIONS

1. The body can generate heat by
A. shivering
B. increasing cellular metabolism
C. strenuous exercise
D. all of the above

2. Which of the following affects the thermal gradient?
A. Ambient air temperature
B. Infrared radiation
C. Relative humidity
D. All of the above

3. Heat loss in the form of infrared rays is known as
A. radiation
B. convection
C. conduction
D. evaporation

4. Heat flows from the skin to the air because of
A. radiation
B. convection
C. conduction
D. evaporation

5. Heat is carried away from the body by a process known as
   A. radiation
   B. convection
   C. conduction
   D. evaporation

6. The key heat regulating center is located in the
   A. thymus gland
   B. thalamus
   C. cerebral cortex
   D. hypothalamus

7. When the body becomes too hot, which of the following happens?
   A. Peripheral vasodilation
   B. Decreased cardiac output
   C. Decreased respiratory rate
   D. Increased thermogenesis

8. When the body becomes too cold, which of the following **DOES NOT** happen?
   A. Sympathetic stimulation
   B. Piloerection
   C. Vasodilation
   D. Thermogenesis

9. Fever differs from hyperthermia in that it
   A. lowers body temperature
   B. is a compensatory mechanism
   C. does not involve the hypothalamus
   D. cooling mechanisms are activated

10. Heat cramps are caused by
   A. a rapid change in extracellular osmolarity
   B. potassium and water losses
   C. increased thermogenesis (shivering)
   D. decreased perfusion of abdominal muscles

11. Heat exhaustion is caused by
   A. increased sodium and water losses
   B. rapid, dangerous elevation of body temperature
   C. peripheral vasoconstriction
   D. increased circulating blood volume

12. Prehospital management of the heat stroke patient includes all of the following **EXCEPT**
   A. rapid cooling
   B. oxygen administration
   C. dopamine IV
   D. IV access

13. In which of the following conditions is prehospital cooling of the fever patient contraindicated?
   A. Altered mental status
   B. Imminent febrile seizures

C. Fever >105°F

D. Fever due to epiglottitis

14. Initial signs of hypothermia include
A. cool, pale skin
B. tachycardia
C. tachypnea
D. all of the above

15. Prehospital management of the frostbite victim includes all of the following **EXCEPT**
A. immersion in 100°–106° F water
B. gently massaging the frozen part
C. elevating the thawed part
D. covering the thawed part with loose sterile dressings

16. The primary cause of death from drowning is
A. acid-base abnormality
B. asphyxia
C. pulmonary edema
D. hemodilution

17. Which of the following factors have an impact on drowning survival?
A. Cleanliness of water
B. Length of submersion
C. Age and health of victim
D. All of the above

18. Which of the following is a result of the mammalian diving reflex?
A. Tachypnea
B. Bradycardia
C. Vasodilation
D. All of the above

19. Prehospital management of the drowning victim includes all of the following **EXCEPT**
A. C-spine management and oxygenation
B. Heimlich maneuver
C. Defibrillation as indicated
D. CPR as indicated

Match the following terms of basic nuclear physics:

20. Protons   **A.** Unstable atoms emitting ionizing radiation

21. Neutrons   **B.** Positively charged particles present in all elements

22. Electrons   **C.** Particles lacking an electrical charge

23. Isotopes   **D.** Negatively charged minute particles

24. Alpha particles   **E.** Low energy particles, easily blocked by clothing

25. Gamma rays   **F.** Dangerous, high energy particles, requires lead shielding

26. Which of the following is an effect of long-term radiation exposure?
A. Decreasing leukocytes
B. Bone marrow damage
C. Birth defects
D. All of the above

27. Which of the following factors will have a major effect on the amount of radiation a person absorbs?
A. Length of time exposed
B. Shielding
C. Distance from the source
D. All of the above

28. According to Boyle's Law, one liter of air at sea level will be compressed to _____ at a depth of 33 feet of water.
A. 1000 ml
B. 500 ml
C. 333 ml
D. 250 ml

29. According to Henry's Law, at 33 feet below the surface the quantity of nitrogen and oxygen dissolved in the tissues will be _____ that at sea level.
A. one-half
B. three times
C. twice
D. four times

30. A person experiencing sinus headache pain, dizzyness, and hearing loss after diving too fast may be suffering from
A. barotrauma
B. eustacian tube rupture
C. middle ear infection
D. all of the above

31. A diver who appears to be intoxicated and takes unecessary risks may be experiencing
A. carbon monoxide poisoning
B. barotrauma
C. the bends
D. nitrogen narcosis

32. A diver who holds his or her breath during ascent may experience
A. air embolism
B. pneumothorax
C. alveoli rupture
D. all of the above

33. A diver who ascends without allowing time for gradual recompression may experience
A. air embolism
B. pneumomediastinum
C. eustacian tube rupture
D. the bends

SCENARIO   Your patient is a 23-year-old construction worker who collapsed on the job. The temperature is 88°F with 78% humidity. He presents on the ground, skin hot, wet, and red. He has no medical history according to his co-workers and there is no Medic-Alert identification. His BP is 90/0, pulse is 120, shallow respirations of 30, lungs clear, chemstrip is 100, axillary temperature is 107°F.

34. This patient is most likely suffering from
   A. heat cramps
   B. heat exhaustion
   C. heat stroke
   D. heat prostation

35. Immediate prehospital management of this patient includes
   A. rapid cooling
   B. oxygenation
   C. IV fluids
   D. vasopressors

36. Glass thermometers are not recommended for prehospital use because
   A. they are easily broken
   B. they do not measure as high or low as necessary
   C. they are difficult to calibrate during long transport times
   D. none of the above

SCENARIO   Your patient is a 38-year-old female who got lost in the woods on a hiking trip. She spent the night in a small cave with overnight temperatures dropping to the mid-twenties. It had rained earlier in the day and she had no time to dry off before settling in the cave. She was found by searchers at around 10 AM the next day. She presents awake, but confused and disoriented. She appears very stiff and her movements are uncoordinated. Her BP is 100/60, pulse is 80, respirations are slow and shallow, skin is cool and pale, chemstrip is 120, axillary temperature is 86°F.

37. This person is suffering from
   A. mild hypothermia
   B. mild-to-moderate hypothermia
   C. moderate-to-severe hypothermia
   D. hyperpyrexia

38. In severe hypothermia, the patient's ECG may show the presence of
   A. delta waves
   B. J waves
   C. coving
   D. ST segment depression

39. Since the nearest hospital is one hour by car, which of the following statements is true regarding the prehospital management of this patient?
   A. Rewarming should not be attempted
   B. Heated oxygen should not be administered

C. External heat should never be applied

D. The patient must be handled gently

40. If the patient loses consciousness and arrests, prehospital management should include all of the following **EXCEPT**

A. CPR

B. defibrillation

C. medication administration

D. heated and humidified oxygen

ANSWERS

1. ANS—D *PEC—864*

The human body can generate heat by shivering, by increasing cellular metabolism, and by strenuous exercise.

2. ANS—D *PEC—865*

Several factors affect a thermal gradient. They include ambient air temperature (the temperature of the surrounding air), infrared radiation (radiation with a wave length longer than that of visible light), and relative humidity (the percentage of water vapor present in the air).

3. ANS—A *PEC—865*

Heat loss in the form of infrared rays is called radiation. All objects not at absolute zero temperature will radiate heat.

4. ANS—C *PEC—865*

Direct contact of the body surface to another cooler object causes the body to loose heat by conduction. Heat flows from higher temperature matter to lower temperature matter. If the ambient air temperature is cooler than the skin temperature, then heat will flow from the skin to the air.

5. ANS—B *PEC—865*

Heat loss to air currents passing over the body is called convection.

6. ANS—D *PEC—866*

The temperature regulating centers are located in the hypothalamus at the base of the brain. This area functions like a thermostat. It produces neurosecretions important in the control of many metabolic activities including temperature regulation.

7. ANS—A *PEC—866*

When the body becomes too hot, it attempts to eliminate body heat through five mechanisms: vasodilation, perspiration, decreased heat production, increased cardiac output, and increased respiratory rate.

8. ANS—C *PEC—867*

When the body becomes too cold, it attempts to preserve heat by engaging the following mechanisms: vasoconstriction, piloerection, increased heat production by shivering, and sympathetic stimulation.

9. ANS—B *PEC—867*

Fever differs from hypothermia in that it is a compensatory mechanism. It is the body's attempt to clear itself of the infectious agent by raising the body temperature.

10. ANS—A   *PEC—869*

Heat cramps are caused primarily by a rapid change in extracellular fluid osmolarity resulting from sodium and water losses. This results in intermittent painful contractions of various skeletal muscles.

11. ANS—A   *PEC—869*

Heat exhaustion results from excessive water and salt loss due to sweating. A deficiency in water and sodium combine to cause electrolyte volume and vasomotor regulatory disturbances.

12. ANS—C   *PEC—870*

Prehospital management of the heat stroke patient includes rapid cooling, oxygen administration, IV access, monitoring ECG, and monitoring core temperatures. Vasopressors and anticholinergic drugs should be avoided.

13. ANS—D   *PEC—871*

Fever should not be treated in the field unless it is extremely high, greater than 105°F, changes in mental status exist, or febrile seizures appear imminent.

14. ANS—D   *PEC—871*

Initial signs of hypothermia are peripheral vasoconstriction with an increase in cardiac output and respiratory rate.

15. ANS—B   *PEC—876*

Prehospital management of the frostbite victim includes immersing the frozen part in water heated to 100°-106°F, elevating the thawed part and covering it with loose sterile dressings.

16. ANS—B   *PEC—877*

Deaths due to drowning and near drowning are primarily caused by asphyxia from airway obstruction in the lungs secondary to the aspirated water or laryngospasm.

17. ANS—D   *PEC—879*

Factors that have an impact on drowning and near drowning survival rates include the cleanliness of the water, the length of time submerged, and the age and general health of the victim.

18. ANS—B   *PEC—879*

When a person dives into cold water he or she reacts to the submersion of the face. This is known as the mammalian diving reflex. In this reflex breathing is inhibited, the heart rate becomes slower, and vasoconstriction develops in the tissues.

19. ANS—B   *PEC—879*

Prehospital management of the drowning victim includes C-spine management, oxygenation, defibrillation, and CPR as indicated.

20. Protons   **B.** Positively charged particles   *PEC—880*
                                    present in all elements

21. Neutrons   **C.** Particles lacking an electrical charge

22. Electrons	**D.**	Negatively charged minute particles
23. Isotopes	**A.**	Unstable atoms emitting ionizing radiation
24. Alpha particles	**E.**	Low energy particles, easily blocked by clothing
25. Gamma rays	**F.**	Dangerous, high energy particles, requires lead shielding

26. ANS—D   *PEC—881*

Cell damage due to inonizing radiation is cumulative over a lifetime. If a person is exposed to inonizing radiation long enough, there will be a decreased number of white blood cells, possible defects in offspring, an increased incidence of cancer, and various degrees of bone marrow damage.

27. ANS—D   *PEC—881*

The amount of radiation received by a person depends upon the source of radiation, the length of time exposed, the distance from the source, and the shielding between the exposed person and the source.

28. ANS—B   *PEC—885*

Air is compressible. Boyle's law states that every 33 feet below the surface you dive, the pressure of gas in your lungs doubles while the volume decreases by one-half. One liter of air at the surface, therefore, is compressed to 500 milliliters at 33 feet below the surface.

29. ANS—C   *PEC—885*

Henry's law states that the amount of gas dissolved in a given volume of fluid is proportional to the pressure of the gas with which it is in equilibrium. Since the body is made up primarily of liquid, gases that are inhaled will be dissolved in the body in proportion to the partial pressure of each breath. The body uses oxygen but it does not use nitrogen. Therefore, the primary gas dissolved in the body is nitrogen because it is inert and not used by the body. At 33 feet below the surface the quantity of oxygen and nitrogen dissolved in the tissues will be twice that at sea level.

30. ANS—A   *PEC—885*

Barotrauma, commonly called "the squeeze," becomes a concern during descent. If the diver cannot equilibrate the pressure between the nasopharynx and the middle ear through the eustachian tube, he or she can experience middle ear pain.

31. ANS—D   *PEC—886*

Major diving emergencies while at the bottom of the dive involve nitrogen narcosis, commonly called "raptures of the deep." This is due to nitrogen's effect on cerebral function.

32. ANS—D   *PEC—886*

The most serious barotrauma can occur if a diver holds his or her breath during the ascent. As a diver ascends, the air in the lungs, which has been compressed, expands. If it's not exhaled, the alveoli may rupture. If this occurs, the result may be structural damage to the lung and air embolism. This may also produce mediastinal and subcutaneous emphysema or pneumothorax.

33. ANS—D   *PEC—886*

A diver who ascends without allowing time for gradual recompression may experience "the bends." This is a condition that develops in divers subjected to rapid reduction of air pressure after ascending to the surface following exposure to compressed air. Nitrogen bubbles enter the tissue spaces in small blood vessels. Bubbles produced by rapid decompression are thought to produce obstruction of blood flow and lead to local ischemia subjecting tissues to anoxia stress.

34. ANS—C   *PEC—870*

This patient is most likely suffering from heat stroke. Heat stroke occurs when the body's hypothalmic temperature regulation is lost causing uncompensated hypothermia which in turn causes cell death and physiologic collapse.

35. ANS—D   *PEC—870*

Immediate prehospital management of the heat stroke patient includes rapid patient cooling, oxygen administration, establishing IVs, monitoring the ECG and core temperature. Vasopressors and anticholinergis drugs are contraindicated since they may inhibit sweating.

36. ANS—B   *PEC—871*

Glass thermometers are not recommended because they usually do not measure above 106°F or below 95°F.

37. ANS—C   *PEC—871*

This patient is suffering from moderate to severe hypothermia.

38. ANS—B   *PEC—873*

The typical hypothermic EKG shows the presence of J waves, also called Osborne waves.

39. ANS—D   *PEC—874*

Rewarming of this patient should be attempted since transportation to the hospital will take more than 15 minutes. External application of heat by warm blankets is a safe and effective means of rewarming the hypothermic patient. Another excellent means of rewarming the hypothermic patient is by administering heated and humidified oxygen. Of course, the hypothermic patient should be moved gently.

40. ANS—C   *PEC—876*

Hospital management of the hypothermic cardiac arrest includes CPR, defibrillation, and administering heated and humidified oxygen.

CHAPTER 29

Emergencies in the Geriatric Patient

1. The fastest growing segment of our population is the elderly because of
   A. a declining birth rate
   B. an absence of major wars and catastrophies
   C. an improved health care system
   D. all of the above

2. Which of the following is an example of age-related body system changes?
   A. Total body water increases
   B. Homeostatic control efficiency reduction
   C. Metabolic rate drops
   D. Total body fat increases

3. Which of the following best describes changes in the respiratory system of elderly patients?
   A. Lung elasticity decreases
   B. Vital capacity decreases
   C. Respiratory muscle strength decreases
   D. All of the above

4. Which of the following best describes changes in the cardiovascular system of elderly patients?
   A. Left ventricular hypertrophy

  B. Conduction system degeneration
  C. Decreasing cardiac output
  D. All of the above

5. Osteoporosis, kyphosis, and spondylolysis are the result of
  A. the demineralizing of bone
  B. fibrosis
  C. decreased nerve conduction velocity
  D. the reduced number of nephrons

6. Which of the following tend to complicate the assessment of the elderly?
  A. The elderly often suffer more than one disease at a time
  B. The primary problem often is different from the chief complaint
  C. The patient's perception of pain may be diminished or absent
  D. All of the above

7. Assessing an elderly patient who presents with poor peripheral pulses, rales, and dependent edema may be difficult because
  A. her presentation is consistent with congestive heart failure
  B. her signs and symptoms may be caused by the aging process
  C. it is often difficult to distinguish acute from chronic problems
  D. all of the above

8. Your patient who complains that the room is spinning, and is nauseated, pale, and sweating, may be suffering from
  A. dementia
  B. delirium
  C. Alzheimer's
  D. vertigo

Match the following causes of syncope with their respective descriptions:

9. ____ Vasodepressor **A.** Temporary stroke

10. ____ Orthostatic **B.** Stokes-Adams syndrome

11. ____ Vasovagal **C.** Rising from a seated or supine position

12. ____ Cardiac **D.** The common faint

13. ____ TIA **E.** Valsalva maneuver

14. Chronic global mental impairment is known as
  A. organic brain syndrome
  B. senile dementia
  C. senility
  D. all of the above

15. Which of the following renders the edlerly susceptible to making medication errors?
  A. Forgetfulness
  B. Limited income
  C. Vision impairment
  D. All of the above

SCENARIO Your patient is an 89-year-old female who presents with multiple bruises. She lives with her son who says she is always falling down and is just generally clumsy. She appears somewhat undernourished and frightened. She cowers when you approach her and reluctantly allows you to inspect her bruises. Her son behaves very strangely toward you and your partner and nervously attempts to explain each bruise. She is incontinent of urine and appears not to have been washed in days. You suspect elderly abuse.

16. In which socioeconomic class is this problem most prevalent?
A. Lower
B. Middle class
C. Wealthy
D. All classes

17. In this case the paramedic should do all of the following EXCEPT
A. Obtain a complete patient and family history
B. Report any suspicions to the ED staff
C. Be honest with her son about your concerns
D. Watch for inconsistencies in stories

SCENARIO Your patient is an 82-year-old woman who presents with some vague complaints about feeling weak and fatigued. She denies any chest pain. She has a long history of cardiac, respiratory, and diabetic problems. She takes a host of medications for each but cannot remember what she took today. In your exam you notice her swollen ankles, weak peripheral pulses, and auscultate some fine bibasilar rales. You suspect she is having a cardiac episode and begin appropriate prehospital management.

18. Which of the following is true regarding this elderly patient?
A. Absence of chest pain does not rule out myocardial infarction
B. Her peripheral edema and rales may be normal findings
C. The first two hours after the onset of symptoms are critical
D. All of the above

19. Atypical presentations of myocardial infarction include
A. dental pain
B. syncope
C. dyspnea
D. all of the above

20. All of the following statements are true regarding the management of the elderly cardiac patient EXCEPT
A. they are treated much the same as the younger patient
B. medication orders may be modified
C. oxygen administration must be carefully monitored
D. fluid administration may be decreased

ANSWERS   **1. ANS—D**   *PEC—894*

The fastest growing segment of our population is the elderly due to a declining birth rate, the absence of major wars and catastrophies, and an improved health care system since World War II.

2. ANS—B   *PEC—895*

In most people of this age group the total amount of body water significantly decreases, the total body fat decreases by as much as 15-30 percent, the metabolic rate remains fairly constant. There is a sharp reduction in the total number of body cells, and more importantly, a progressive reduction in the efficiency of the body's homeostatic system.

3. ANS—D   *PEC—896*

The effects of aging on the respiratory system include increased chest wall stiffness, loss of lung elasticity, increased air trapping, reduced strength and endurance of the respiratory muscles, decreasing vital capacity, maximum breathing capacity, and maximum oxygen uptake.

4. ANS—D   *PEC—896*

Changes in the cardiovascular system include left ventricular hypertrophy, fibrosis in the heart and peripheral vascular system, conductive system degeneration, and decreased cardiac output.

5. ANS—A   *PEC—896*

Osteoporosis, kyphosis, and spondylolysis are the result of the demineralizing of bone. This results in softening of bone tissue.

6. ANS—D   *PEC—897*

It is difficult to assess the elderly because they often suffer more than one disease at a time. Their primary problem is often different from the chief complaint and their perception of pain may be diminished or absent.

7. ANS—D   *PEC—897*

Assessing elderly patients who present with poor peripheral pulses, rales, and edema may be difficult because their presentation is consistent with congestive heart failure, and yet their signs and symptoms may be caused by the simple aging process. It is often difficult to distinguish the acute from the chronic problem.

8. ANS—D   *PEC—904*

Vertigo is a specific sensation of motion perceived by the patient as spinning or whirling. It is often accompanied by sweating, pallor, nausea, and vomiting.

9. ____ Vasodepressor   **D.** The common faint   *PEC—902*

10. ____ Orthostatic   **C.** Rising from a seated or supine position

11. ____ Vasovagal   **E.** Valsalva maneuver

12. ____ Cardiac   **B.** Stokes-Adams syndrome

13. ____ TIA   **A.** Temporary stroke

14. ANS—D   *PEC—905*

Dementia is a chronic, global mental impairment often progressive or irreversible usually due to underlying neurological disease. This mental deterioration is often called organic brain syndrome, senile dementia, or senility.

15. ANS—D   *PEC—908*

Underdosing and overdosing of medication is very common in the elderly. It may be due to confusion, vision impairment, forgetfulness, or limited income.

16. ANS—D   *PEC—909*

Abuse of the elderly knows no social economic bounds. It occurs in all classes of our society and is a major health and social problem.

17. ANS—C   *PEC—909*

In cases where you suspect geriatric abuse, you should obtain a complete patient and family history and watch for inconsistencies in the stories. You should report any suspicions to the ED staff and always avoid confrontations with the family.

18. ANS—D   *PEC—902*

In this case, the absence of chest pain does not rule out myocardial infarction because many elderly patients suffer silent myocardial infarctions. Her peripheral edema in rales may be normal findings of the aging process and as in all cardiac patients, the first two hours after the onset of symptoms are the most critical.

19. ANS—D   *PEC—902*

Atypical presentations of myocardial infarction include dental pain, syncope, dyspnea, confusion, neck pain, epigastric pain, and fatigue.

20. ANS—C   *PEC—903*

Managing the elderly cardiac patient is somewhat the same as managing the younger cardiac patient with a few differences. Medication orders may be modified and fluid administration may be decreased based on the presence of congestive heart failure, liver disease, and other metabolic problems.

CHAPTER 30

Emergencies in the Pediatric Patient

QUESTIONS

1. The leading cause of death in the 1-15 year age group is/are
A. accidents
B. respiratory illness
C. SIDS
D. congenital problems

2. The age group most obsessed with monsters and mutilation is
A. 1-3 years
B. 3-5 years
C. 5-12 years
D. 12-15 years

3. A sunken anterior fontanelle may indicate
A. increased intracranial pressure
B. meningitis
C. epidural hematoma
D. dehydration

4. As a rule, as a child gets older
A. the BP falls and the pulse rate rises
B. the BP rises and the pulse rate falls
C. the BP and pulse rates fall
D. the BP and pulse rates rise

5. Which of the following airways is recommended for pediatric use?
   A. Esophageal Obturator Airway (EOA)
   B. Nasopharyngeal Airways
   C. Pharyngeaotracheal Lumen Airway (PTL)
   D. None of the above

6. The narrowest portion of the upper pediatric airway is at the
   A. larynx
   B. vocal cords
   C. cricoid ring
   D. arytenoids

7. Pop-off valves should be functional when ventilating the pediatric patient
   A. to avoid over inflation of the lungs
   B. to avoid causing a pneumothorax
   C. to avoid barotrauma to the lungs
   D. none of the above

8. The commonly accepted age limit for attempting an intraosseous infusion is
   A. 3 years old
   B. 5 years old
   C. 7 years old
   D. none of the above

9. Verifying proper placement of an intraosseous needle includes
   A. noting a lack of resistance
   B. the needle standing upright
   C. free flow of infusion without infiltration
   D. all of the above

10. The initial dose for defibrillation in the pediatric patient is
   A. 1 j/kg
   B. 2 j/kg
   C. 4 j/kg
   D. 200 j

11. A 3-year-old child who burns both legs and arms has burned approximately _____% of his entire body surface area.
   A. 54
   B. 45
   C. 72
   D. 36

12. Which of the following children may be at a higher risk for child abuse?
   A. Handicapped children
   B. Twin child
   C. Premature child
   D. All of the above

13. Which of the following are classic characteristics of a child abuser?
   A. Parent who spends majority of time with child
   B. Parent who was abused as child

C. Parent experiencing financial or marital stress
D. All of the above

14. Prehospital management of the abused child includes all of the following **EXCEPT**
A. treating all injuries
B. elliciting a complete history from child and parents
C. allowing parent to drive child to hospital
D. reporting your findings to the emergency department staff

15. Which of the following statements regarding febrile seizures is true?
A. They usually occur between the ages of 6 months and 1 year
B. They are caused by extremely high temperatures
C. They are caused by a sudden increase in temperature
D. The patient usually does not need to be transported

16. Which of the following statements is true regarding SIDS?
A. It usually occurs between the ages of 1 year and 3 years
B. Death usually occurs during sleep
C. It is usually caused by external suffocation
D. All children are at equal risk

SCENARIO Your patient is a 2-month-old who presents lethargic and febrile. His mother says that he has been ill with upper respiratory congestion for two days. He has not eaten well and he generally appears to be very ill. His anterior fontanelles are sunken, he is tachycardic, tachypneic, with a four second capillary refill.

17. You should suspect _____ until proven otherwise.
A. Reye's syndrome
B. Down's syndrome
C. meningitis
D. bronchiolitis

18. His vital signs indicate that this patient
A. is in respiratory failure
B. is in shock
C. has increased intracranial pressure
D. none of the above

19. Prehospital management should include oxygen and
A. IV Mannitol
B. 20mg/kg IV fluid challenge
C. IV antibiotics
D. the pneumatic antishock garment

SCENARIO Your patient is a 7-year-old who presents with severe nausea and vomiting. His mother says he has had the flu for two days and that she gave him aspirin to lower his fever. He exhibits some combative behavior and appears restless. He has rapid, deep respirations and sluggish pupils. His pulse rate is 60, BP is 150/80.

20. Judging from his history and physical finding, you should suspect
  A. asthma
  B. meningitis
  C. sepsis
  D. Reye's syndrome

21. His physical exam shows the presence of
  A. shock
  B. poisoning
  C. vaso-vagal episode
  D. increased intracranial pressure

SCENARIO Your patient is a 3-year-old who presents with a sudden onset of severe difficulty in breathing. She has not been ill and had been playing with friends at the time of onset. She presents afebrile with inspiratory stridor, a weak cough, and ashen skin.

22. You should suspect
  A. foreign body obstruction
  B. croup
  C. epiglottitis
  D. asthma

23. Initial prehospital management of this patient includes
  A. back blows
  B. abdominal thrusts
  C. leaving the patient alone
  D. encouraging the patient to cough

24. Further management of this patient may include
  A. direct layngoscopy
  B. removal with Magill forceps
  C. cricothyrotomy
  D. all of the above

SCENARIO Your patient is a 5-year-old who presents sitting forward using all accessory muscles to breathe. He has inspiratory stridor, retractions, a sore throat, and drools. He is febrile and has been ill for almost a week prior to this incident.

25. In this patient, you should suspect
  A. foreign body obstruction
  B. croup
  C. epiglottitis
  D. asthma

26. Initial prehospital management of this patient includes
  A. racemic epinephrine
  B. direct layngoscopy

    C. Heimlich maneuver

    D. none of the above

27. If the patient totally occludes his airway, you should immediately

    A. deliver 5 abdominal thrusts

    B. perform bag-valve-mask ventilation

    C. inject 0.03 mg/kg epinephrine 1: 1000 SC

    D. none of the above

SCENARIO Your patient is an 8-month-old child who presents with difficulty in breathing. She has diffuse expiratory wheezing, retractions, and uses accessory muscles to move air. She is tachypneic and tachycardic. She is warm and has been ill since yesterday.

28. In this patient you should suspect

    A. asthma

    B. bronchitis

    C. bronchiolitis

    D. croup

29. Signs that this patient is in imminent respiratory arrest would include

    A. slowing of the respiratory rate

    B. decrease in the respiratory effort

    C. decrease in breath sounds

    D. all of the above

30. Prehospital management of this patient should include

    A. oxygen

    B. albuterol via nebulizer

    C. sitting child upright

    D. all of the above

SCENARIO Your patient is a 4-year-old who presents listless and appears very ill. She has a decreased level of consciousness and responds only to loud voices. Her mother says she has had diarrhea for two days and has not been able to keep food or drink down. She has tenting, dry mucous membranes, tachycardia, and delayed capillary refill.

31. From this patient's presentation, you should suspect

    A. respiratory failure

    B. severe dehydration

    C. pulmonary edema

    D. respiratory infection

32. Prehospital management should include oxygen and

    A. 20mg/kg IV fluid challenge

    B. 40 mg furosemide IV

    C. IV antibiotics

    D. albuterol via nebulizer

ANSWERS   **1. ANS—A**   *PEC—915*

Accidents of all types are the leading cause of death between the ages of 1 and 15 years.

2. ANS—B   *PEC—915*

Children in the 3-5 age group have vivid imaginations and may see monsters as part of their world. During this stage of development children have a fear of mutilation and may view treatment procedures as hostile.

3. ANS—D   *PEC—919*

The anterior fontanelle should be inspected in all infants. It should be level with the surface of the skull or slightly sunken and it may pulsate. With dehydration the anterior fontanelle may often fall below the level of the skull and appear sunken.

4. ANS—B   *PEC—919*

As a rule, as a child gets older the blood pressure rises and the pulse rate falls.

5. ANS—B   *PEC—945*

Certain airways in pediatrics are contraindicated because of variations in airway size in children. Avoid esophageal obturator airways, pharyngealtracheal lumen airways, and esophageal combitubes. Also, nasopharyngeal airways are discouraged because young children have rather large adenoidal tissue and insertion of an NPA can lacerate these tissues causing bleeding into the airway.

6. ANS—C   *PEC—945*

The narrowest portion of the upper pediatric airway is at the cricoid ring. For this reason uncuffed endotracheal tubes should be used for all children under the age of eight because the cricoid ring acts as an anatomical cuff holding the tube in place, securing the airway.

7. ANS—D   *PEC—946*

Pediatric bag-valve-masks should not contain pressure pop-off valves. If one exists, it should be disengaged. The reason is that higher pressures may be needed to ventilate the pediatric patient.

8. ANS—B   *PEC—946*

Indications for intraosseous infusion include an unresponsive child less than five years of age in shock or cardiac arrest, after unsuccessful attempts at peripheral IV insertion. In children over the age of five, the bones become more solid.

9. ANS—D   *PEC—946*

Placement of the needle into the marrow cavity can be determined by noting a lack of resistance if the needle passes through the bony cortex. Other indications include the needle standing upright without support, the ability to aspirate bone marrow into a syringe, or free flow of the infusion without infiltration into the subcutaneous tissues.

10. ANS—B   *PEC—951*

The initial dose for defibrillation in pediatric patients is 2 joules per kilogram. Perform all subsequent defibrillation attempts at 4 joules per kilogram.

11. ANS—A   *PEC—923*

Estimation of the burn surface is slightly different for children. When using the rule of nines to calculate the percentage of burns in infants and small children, each leg is worth 13.5% while the head is worth 18%. For this patient who burned both legs and arms, the body surface area adds up to 54%.

12. ANS—D   *PEC—923*

There are several characteristics common to abused children. Often they are seen as special and different from others. Also, premature infants or twins, children less than five years of age, handicapped children, uncommunicative children, boys, and children of the wrong sex are at higher risk.

13. ANS—D   *PEC—924*

The child abuser can come from any geographic, religious, ethnic, occupational, educational, or socioeconomic group. However, people who abuse children tend to share certain characteristics. The abuser is usually a parent or someone in the role of a parent. When the mother spends most time with the child, she is the parent most frequently identified as the abuser. Most child abusers were abused as children. Common crises (financial stress, marital or relationship stress, and physical illness in a parent or child) may precipitate abuse.

14. ANS—C   *PEC—926*

The prehospital management of the abused child includes: appropriately treating the injuries, protecting the child from further abuse, notifying the proper authorities, obtaining as much information as possible in a non-judgmental manner, documenting all findings or statements in the patient report.

15. ANS—C   *PEC—927*

Febrile seizures occur as a result of a sudden increase in body temperature. They seem related to the rate at which the body temperature increases, not to the degree of fever.

16. ANS—B   *PEC—940*

Sudden infant death syndrome usually occurs in children between the ages of one month and one year during sleep. It is not caused by any type of external suffocation. Certain children (males, infants with a low birth weight, children of young mothers, from lower socioeconomic groups) are predisposed to SIDS.

17. ANS—C   *PEC—928*

Documented fever in a child less than three months of age is considered meningitis until proven otherwise.

18. ANS—B   *PEC—936*

The patient's vital signs, sunken anterior fontanels, tachycardia, tachypnea, and delayed capillary refill all indicate shock.

19. ANS—B   *PEC—936*

Prehospital management of this patient should include oxygen and a fluid challenge of 20 milliliters per kilogram of IV crystalloids (normal saline, Lactated Ringer's).

20. ANS—D   *PEC—929*

Judging from this patient's history of two-day flu and aspirin administration and the physical findings which indicate increased intracranial pressure and combative behavior, you should suspect Reye's syndrome.

21. ANS—D *PEC—929*

The physical exam shows the presence of rapid respirations, sluggish pupils, bradycardia, and hypertension. This patient shows the presence of increased cranial pressure.

22. ANS—A *PEC—930*

Any afebrile child who presents with a sudden onset of stridor without previous history of illness, should be suspected as having a foreign body obstruction.

23. ANS—B *PEC—930*

Initial prehospital management of this patient includes delivering five abdominal thrusts.

24. ANS—D *PEC—930*

Further management of this patient may include direct laryngoscopy and removal of the foreign body with Magill forceps and, as a last resort, needle cricothyrotomy.

25. ANS—C *PEC—932*

Your 5-year-old patient who sits forward, drooling, presenting with stridor, fever, and illness should be suspected of having epiglottitis.

26. ANS—D *PEC—933*

Initial prehospital management of this patient includes placing a child in a position of comfort and administering humidified oxygen by face mask or blow-by. Direct visualization of the larynx may cause laryngospasm and is contraindicated.

27. ANS—B *PEC—933*

If the patient totally closes his airway (usually from laryngospasm), immediately perform bag-valve-mask ventilation.

28. ANS—C *PEC—933*

In this patient, who is less than one-year-old presenting with wheezing and difficulty breathing, you should suspect bronchiolitis.

29. ANS—D *PEC—933*

Signs that a pediatric patient is in imminent respiratory arrest include slowing of the respiratory rate, a decrease in the respiratory effort, and a decrease in breath sounds.

30. ANS—D *PEC—933*

Prehospital management of this patient should include oxygen administration, sitting the child upright, and administering albuterol via nebulizer.

31. ANS—B *PEC—936*

This child who presents with dry mucous membranes, poor skin turgor, tachycardia, and delayed capillary refill is suspected of having severe dehydration.

32. ANS—A *PEC—936*

Prehospital management of this patient should include oxygen and 20 milliliters per kilogram of IV crystalloids (normal saline, Lactated Ringer's).

DIVISION 5—OB/GYN, NEONATAL

CHAPTER 31

Gynechological Emergencies

QUESTIONS

1. Fertilization normally occurs in the
    A. ovaries
    B. fallopian tubes
    C. uterus
    D. vagina

2. The uterine lining that sloughs off during the menstrual period is the
    A. perineum
    B. endometrium
    C. labia minora
    D. menarche

3. The function of the ovaries is to produce
    A. estrogen
    B. progesterone
    C. eggs for reproduction
    D. all of the above

4. A fertilized egg normally implants on the
    A. uterine wall
    B. cervix
    C. perineum
    D. urethra

5. The neck of the uterus that dilates to allow passage of the baby is the
A. perineum
B. fallopian opening
C. cervix
D. endometrium

6. The area surrounding the vagina that sometimes tears during childbirth is the
A. perineum
B. endometrium
C. urethra
D. cervix

7. A woman's gravidity refers to her number of
A. pregnancies
B. viable deliveries
C. abortions
D. cesarean sections

8. A woman's parity refers to her number of
A. pregnancies
B. viable deliveries
C. abortions
D. cesarean sections

9. The beginning of menses is called
A. menopause
B. menarche
C. ovulation
D. menstruation

10. Physical examination of the gynechological patient includes all of the following EXCEPT
A. palpating for masses
B. inspecting for distention and guarding
C. asking about tenderness
D. performing an internal vaginal exam

11. Common complications of pelvic inflammatory disease include
A. sepsis
B. ectopic pregnancies
C. pelvic organ adhesions
D. all of the above

12. The most common site for ectopic pregnancies is
A. the uterus
B. a fallopian tube
C. the cervix
D. the abdomen

13. Prehospital management of female gynechological trauma includes
A. vaginal packing

B. IV D$_5$W run wide open

C. direct pressure on the external genitalia

D. none of the above

14. Which of the following statements is true regarding sexual assault?

    A. Most victims are female

    B. Paramedics should not question the victim about the incident in the field

    C. Paramedics should not perform physical examination of the genitalia

    D. All of the above

15. Which of the following statements is true regarding the preserving of evidence in sexual assault cases?

    A. Place all clothing items in the same bag

    B. Use plastic bags for blood-soaked articles

    C. Do not allow the patient to clean her fingernails

    D. Clean the patient's wounds

ANSWERS

1. ANS—B   *PEC—954*

The fallopian tubes are hollow tubes that transport the egg from the ovary to the uterus. Fertilization usually occurs in a fallopian tube.

2. ANS—B   *PEC—956*

The endometrium is the lining of the uterus. Each month under the influence of estrogen and progesterone, the endometrium builds up in preparation of a fertilized ovum. If fertilization does not occur, the lining simply sloughs off. The sloughing off of the uterine lining is referred to as the menstrual period.

3. ANS—D   *PEC—954*

The ovaries are the female gonads. They produce estrogen, progesterone, and eggs for reproduction.

4. ANS—A   *PEC—954*

The uterus is a small pear-shaped organ that connects with the vagina. The fertilized egg normally implants on the uterine wall.

5. ANS—C   *PEC—956*

The cervix or neck of the uterus is visible through the vagina. During labor the cervix dilates from its closed state to a diameter of approximately 10 centimeters or more, allowing for passage of the baby.

6. ANS—A   *PEC—956*

The perineum is the area surrounding the vagina and anus. This area is sometimes torn during childbirth.

7. ANS—A   *PEC—958*

A woman's gravidity refers to her number of pregnancies. A nulligravida has never been pregnant. A primigravida is pregnant for the first time. A multigravida has been pregnant more than once.

Common Obstetrical Terminology

Term	Meaning
antepartum	the time interval prior to delivery of the fetus
postpartum	the time interval after delivery of the fetus
prenatal	the time interval prior to birth, synonymous with antepartum
natal	literally means birth
gravidity	the number of times a woman has been pregnent
primigravida	a woman who is pregnant for the first time
multigravida	a woman who has been pregnant more than once
nulligravida	a woman who has not been pregnant
parity	the number of times a woman has delivered a viable fetus
primipara	a woman who has delivered her first child
multipara	a woman who has delivered more than one baby
nullipara	a woman who has yet to deliver her first child
grand multiparity	a woman who has delivered at least seven babies

The gravidity and parity of a woman is expressed in the following convention: G_4P_2. "G" refers to the gravidity, and "P" refers to the parity.

8. ANS—B   *PEC—958*

A woman's parity refers to her number of viable deliveries. A nulliparous has never delivered a viable infant. A primiparous has delivered one child. A multiparous has delivered many babies.

9. ANS—B   *PEC—957*

The female undergoes a monthly hormonal cycle that prepares the uterus to receive a fertilized egg. A girl's menses or menstrual period usually begins between 12- and 14-years-old. The beginning of the menses is called menarche.

10. ANS—D   *PEC—957*

Physical examination of the gynecological patients should be limited to taking a good history, and palpating for masses, distention, and guarding. Never perform an internal vaginal exam in the field.

11. ANS—D   *PEC—959*

Pelvic inflammatory disease is an infection of the female reproductive tract. Common complications of PID include sepsis, pelvic organ adhesions, and future ectopic pregnancies.

12. ANS—B   *PEC—960*

Ectopic pregnancy is the implantation of a growing fetus in a place where it does not belong. The most common site is within a fallopian tube.

13. ANS—C   *PEC—961*

Prehospital management of female gynecological trauma includes: managing a laceration by direct pressure on the external genitalia, maintaining intravascular blood volume by starting an IV of Lactated Ringer's and applying antishock trousers. Never pack the vagina with any material or dressing regardless of the severity of the bleeding.

14. ANS—D   *PEC—961*

Sexual assault is one of the fastest growing crimes in the United States. Most victims are female and know their assailants. The victim should not be questioned about the incident in the field since it is not important from the standpoint of prehospital care to determine whether penetration took place. A medic should never perform a physical examination of the genitalia in a possible sexual abuse case.

15. ANS—C   *PEC—961*

There are certain things a paramedic can do to preserve physical evidence in a sexual assault case. These include: not using plastic bags for blood stained articles, bagging each item separately if they must be bagged, handling clothing as little as possible if at all, not allowing the patient to comb her hair or clean her fingernails, not allowing to change her clothes, bath, or douche before the medical exam, and not cleaning wounds if at all possible.

CHAPTER 32

Obstetrical Emergencies

QUESTIONS

1. Which of the following events occurs 14 days before the beginning of the next menstrual period?
A. Ovulation
B. Fertilization
C. Implantation
D. Effacement

2. Fertilization normally occurs in the
A. uterus
B. placenta
C. cervical opening
D. fallopian tubes

3. The umbilical cord contains
A. one artery and one vein
B. two arteries and two veins
C. one artery and two veins
D. two arteries and one vein

4. The estimated date of confinement (EDC) refers to
A. the date of conception
B. the due date
C. when the mother will be admitted to the hospital
D. the date of implantation

5. Immediately following birth, which of the following happens?
   A. The ductus arteriosis closes, diverting blood to the lungs
   B. The ductus venosus closes, stopping blood flow from the placenta
   C. The foramen ovale closes, stopping blood flow between the atria
   D. All of the above

6. A woman with a fundal height of 18 centimeters, the pregnancy is approximately
   A. 6 weeks
   B. 9 weeks
   C. 18 weeks
   D. 36 weeks

7. Which of the following statements is true regarding vital sign changes in the pregnant woman?
   A. The blood presure rises and the pulse rate falls
   B. The blood pressure falls and the pulse rate rises
   C. The blood pressure and pulse rise
   D. The blood pressure and pulse fall

8. The bulging of the baby's head past the opening of the vagina is called
   A. effacement
   B. primipara
   C. prolapsing
   D. crowning

Match the following types of abortion with their respective definitions:

9. ____ Spontaneous   **A.** Abortion performed to save the mother's life

10. ____ Incomplete   **B.** Some fetal tissue passed

11. ____ Criminal   **C.** Miscarraige

12. ____ Therapeutic   **D.** Abortion performed by non-licensed person

13. ____ Elective   **E.** Abortion requested by mother

14. The first stage of labor begins with
   A. the crowning of the infant's head
   B. dilation of the cervix
   C. delivery of the baby
   D. the onset of uterine contractions

15. The second stage of labor begins with
   A. the crowning of the infant's head
   B. dilation of the cervix
   C. delivery of the baby
   D. the onset of uterine contractions

16. The third stage of labor begins with
   A. the crowning of the infant's head
   B. dilation of the cervix
   C. delivery of the baby
   D. the onset of uterine contractions

17. Complete dilation of the cervix is considered to be
A. 5 cm
B. 10 cm
C. 15 cm
D. 20 cm

18. Management of a patient with postpartum hemorrhage includes all of the following EXCEPT
A. fundal massage
B. pitocin IV
C. PASG
D. vaginal packing

19. Which of the following distinguishes preeclampsia from eclampsia?
A. Vaginal bleeding
B. Visual disturbances
C. Grand mal seizures
D. Peripheral edema

20. Magnesium IV may be ordered for which of the following situations?
A. Lower abdominal pain
B. Postpartum hemorrhage
C. Eclamptic seizures
D. Preterm labor pains

SCENARIO Your patient is a 19-year-old woman who presents with severe lower abdominal pain and vaginal bleeding. She claims she is not pregnant but has not had her period for at least 7 weeks. She also complains of weakness, nausea, and vomiting. She admits to being sexually active with multiple partners. She was seen in the ED for several cases of PID in the past two years. Her BP is 90/60, pulse rate 110, respirations 24, skin cool and clammy.

21. You should suspect
A. abruptio placenta
B. placenta previa
C. PID
D. ruptured ectopic pregnancy

22. Her problem was caused by
A. the premature separation of the placenta from the uterine wall
B. the uterus covering the cervical opening
C. an inflamed appendix
D. implantation of the fertilized ovum in a fallopian tube

23. Management of this patient includes all of the following EXCEPT
A. IV fluids
B. vaginal packing
C. PASG
D. high flow oxygen

SCENARIO Your patient is a 26-year-old 30-week pregnant patient who complains of severe tearing abdominal pain and some minor vaginal bleeding. Upon palpation, her abdomen is very tender and her uterus seems to be tightly contracted. Fetal heart tones are absent. She is multigravida, but nullipara.

24. You should suspect
  A. abruptio placenta
  B. placenta previa
  C. miscarraige
  D. ectopic pregnancy

25. Her problem was caused by
  A. the premature separation of the placenta from the uterine wall
  B. the uterus covering the cervical opening
  C. a spontaneous abortion
  D. implantation of the fertilized ovum in a fallopian tube

26. This patient's pregnancy history includes
  A. one pregnancy and one birth
  B. many pregnancies and one birth
  C. one pregnancy and no births
  D. many pregnancies and no births

27. Management of this patient includes all of the following EXCEPT
  A. IV fluids
  B. vaginal packing
  C. PASG
  D. high-flow oxygen

SCENARIO Your patient is a 30-year-old multigravida in her 30th week. She presents with bright red vaginal bleeding but denies any abdominal pain. Her uterus is soft and feels "out of place." Her problem began following sexual intercourse with her husband.

28. You should suspect
  A. abruptio placenta
  B. placenta previa
  C. miscarraige
  D. ectopic pregnancy

29. Her problem was caused by
  A. the premature separation of the placenta from the uterine wall
  B. the uterus covering the cervical opening
  C. a spontaneous abortion
  D. implantation of the fertilized ovum in a fallopian tube

30. Management of this patient includes all of the following EXCEPT
  A. IV fluids
  B. vaginal exam
  C. PASG
  D. high-flow oxygen

ANSWERS

1. ANS—A *PEC—966*

Fourteen days before the beginning of the next menstrual period, the ovum is released from the ovary into the abdominal cavity. This is known as ovulation.

2. ANS—D *PEC—966*

Fertilization is the combination of the female ovum and the male spermatozoa. This usually takes place in a fallopian tube.

3. ANS—D *PEC—966*

The placenta is attached to the developing fetus by the umbilical cord. This cord normally contains two arteries and one vein.

4. ANS—B *PEC—968*

The estimated date of confinement (EDC) is the mother's due date.

5. ANS—D *PEC—968*

The fetal circulation changes immediately at birth. As soon as the baby takes a breath the ambient pressure in the lungs decreases dramatically. Because of this pressure change, the ductus arteriosus closes, diverting blood to the lungs. In addition, the ductus venosus closes, stopping blood flow from the placenta. The foramen ovale also closes from the result of pressure changes in the heart which stops blood flow from the right to the left atrium.

6. ANS—C *PEC—971*

The fundal height is the distance from the pubis to the top of the uterine fundus. Each centimeter of fundal height roughly corresponds to a week of gestation. Therefore, a women of a fundal height of 18 centimeters has been pregnant approximately 18 weeks.

7. ANS—B *PEC—971*

Because of normal changes occurring in the cardiovascular system of the pregnant women, her blood pressure tends to be lower during pregnancy and the pulse rate tends to be faster.

8. ANS—D *PEC—971*

Crowning is the bulging of the fetal head past the opening of the vagina during a contraction. It is an indication of an impending delivery.

9.___ Spontaneous   **C.** Miscarraige   *PEC—974*

10.___ Incomplete   **B.** Some fetal tissue passed

11.___ Criminal   **D.** Abortion performed by non-licensed person

12.___ Therapeutic   **A.** Abortion performed to save the mother's life

13.___ Elective   **E.** Abortion requested by mother

14. ANS—D *PEC—981*

The first stage of labor begins with the onset of uterine contractions and ends with complete dilation of the cervix. It lasts approximately eight hours in nulliparouswomen and five hours in multiparous women.

15. ANS—B *PEC—982*

The second stage of labor begins with complete dilation of the cervix and ends with delivery of the fetus. In the nulliparous patient the second stage lasts approximately 50 minutes and in multiparous women it lasts approximately 20 minutes.

16. ANS—C   *PEC—982*

The third stage of labor begins with delivery of the fetus and ends with the delivery of the placenta. Delivery of the placenta usually occurs within 30 minutes after birth.

17. ANS—B   *PEC—982*

Complete dilation of the cervix is considered to be 10 centimeters.

18. ANS—D   *PEC—991*

Postpartum hemorrhage is the loss of 500 millimeters or more of blood in the first 24 hours following delivery. Prehospital management of the post-partum hemorrhage patient includes: administering oxygen and beginning external fundal massage, administering large bore IVs of normal saline or Lactated Ringer's, and applying anti-shock trousers. Never pack the vagina.

19. ANS—C   *PEC—978*

Eclampsia is the most serious manifestation of hypertensive disorders of pregnancy. It is characterized by grand mal seizure activity.

20. ANS—C   *PEC—978*

Magnesium sulfate may be ordered for eclamptic seizures.

21. ANS—D   *PEC—975*

Ectopic pregnancy is difficult to diagnosis in the field. However, any woman of childbearing age who presents with lower abdominal pain, vaginal bleeding, and a late menstrual period should be suspected of having a ruptured ectopic pregnancy.

22. ANS—D   *PEC—975*

Ectopic pregnancy is the implantation of a fertilized ovum outside of the uterus, most commonly in a fallopian tube. The ovum however can implant anywhere else in the abdominal cavity.

23. ANS—B   *PEC—975*

Management of the patient with a suspected ruptured ectopic pregnancy includes: treating for shock, IV fluids, pneumatic anti-shock garment, and high-flow oxygen.

24. ANS—A   *PEC—975*

Any pregnant patient in her third trimester who complains of tearing abdominal pain and vaginal bleeding should be suspected of having an abruptio placenta.

25. ANS—A   *PEC—976*

Abruptio placenta is the premature separation of the placenta from the wall of the uterus. The separation can be either partial or complete.

26. ANS—D   *PEC—976*

This patient is multigravida and nullipara. Gravida refers to her number of pregnancies which are many. Her parity refers to her number of viable births which were none.

27. ANS—B   *PEC—977*

Management of this patient includes IV fluids, pneumatic anti-shock garment (legs only), high-flow oxygen, generally treating for shock.

28. ANS—B   *PEC—977*

This patient probably has placenta previa. Her history of third-trimester pregnancy, multigravida, and bleeding following intercourse is consistent with this diagnosis.

29. ANS—B   *PEC—977*

Placenta previa is the attachment of the placenta very low in the uterus so that it partially or completely covers the internal cervical opening.

30. ANS—B   *PEC—977*

Treatment for this patient is aimed at treating for shock: IV fluids, pneumatic anti-shock garment, high-flow oxygen.

CHAPTER 33

Emergency Care of the Neonate

QUESTIONS

1. Which of the following is recommended immediately following delivery of the infant?
   A. Position the baby, head down, at the level of the vagina
   B. Suction the mouth, then the nose
   C. Dry the baby off
   D. All of the above

2. Which of the following is recommended practice regarding the umbilical cord?
   A. Milk the cord toward the baby
   B. Milk the cord toward the mother
   C. Clamp and cut the cord shortly after delivery
   D. Disregard the cord until the placenta delivers

3. The normal respiratory rate of the neonate should be _____ breaths per minute.
   A. 10-20
   B. 20-40
   C. 40-60
   D. 60-100

4. A pulse rate of less than 100 beats per minute in the newborn infant
   A. is normal after 2-3 minutes postpartum
   B. indicates an infant in distress

      C. requires immediate atropine administration

      D. requires aggressive fluid therapy

5. Which of the following statements is true regarding the APGAR score?

      A. It should be calculated at 1 and 5 minutes after delivery

      B. An infant with a score of 3 requires immediate resuscitation

      C. Scores in the 7-10 range indicate a normal infant

      D. All of the above

6. The presence of meconium at birth requires immediate

      A. bag-valve mask ventilation

      B. suctioning of the trachea

      C. stimulation of the baby to breathe

      D. cardiopulmonary resuscitation

7. Which of the following statements is true regarding neonatal suctioning?

      A. Normal suctioning should be performed by bulb syringe or Delee trap

      B. Suctioning should last no longer than 10 seconds

      C. Meconium should be suctioned through an endotracheal tube

      D. All of the above

8. Which of the following is **NOT** part of the first step of the inverted pyramid?

      A. Oxygen administration

      B. Tactile stimulation

      C. Drying and warming

      D. Positioning

9. An infant's best indicator of distress is the

      A. respiratory effort

      B. heart rate

      C. cardiac rhythm

      D. blood pressure

10. If the infant presents with cyanosis after performing step 1 of the inverted pyramid, you should

      A. administer blow-by oxygen

      B. perform bag-valve-mask ventilation

      C. begin CPR

      D. insert an endotracheal tube

11. If the heart rate is less than 100, or the infant is still cyanotic after performing step 2, you should

      A. administer blow-by oxygen

      B. perform bag-valve-mask ventilation

      C. begin CPR

      D. insert an endotracheal tube

12. If the infant's heart rate is less than 80 after performing steps 1-3, you should

      A. administer atropine

      B. perform chest compressions

    C. insert an endotracheal tube

    D. administer epinephrine

13. The infant's heart rate can best be checked by

    A. auscultating the heart at the apex

    B. feeling the umbilical cord

    C. palpating the brachial pulse

    D. all of the above

14. Which of the following is true regarding neonatal resuscitation?

    A. Pop-off valves on bag-valve devices should be disengaged

    B. Cuffed ET tubes should be used on all neonates

    C. Chest compressions should be performed on the midsternum

    D. All of the above

15. Fill in the steps of the inverted pyramid:

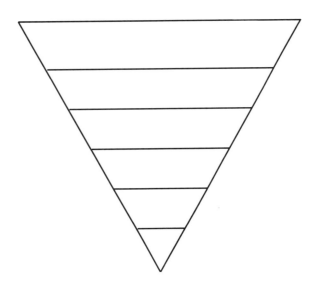

ANSWERS   **1. ANS—D**   *PEC—998*

Routine care of the newborn infant is the first step of the inverted pyramid. This step includes drying and warming the baby; positioning the baby head-down at the level of the vagina; suctioning the mouth, then the nose; and performing tactile stimulation if necessary.

2. ANS—C   *PEC—999*

After you have stabilized the neonate's airway and prevented heat loss, clamp and cut the umbilical cord. Apply the umbilical clamps within 30-45 seconds after birth. Place the first clamp approximately 10 cm from the neonate; place the second clamp approximately 5 cm distal from the first clamp, then cut the cord between the two clamps. After the cord is cut, inspect it periodically to make sure there is no additional bleeding.

3. ANS—C   *PEC—999*

The normal respiratory rate of the neonate should be 40-60 breaths per minute.

4. ANS—B   *PEC—999*

The heart rate is the critical component of neonatal resuscitation. A pulse rate of less than 100 beats per minute in the newborn indicates an infant in distress.

5. ANS—D *PEC—999*

As soon as possible assign the neonate an APGAR score. Do this at one and five minutes after birth. A score of 7-10 indicates an active and vigorous neonate that requires only routine care. Neonates with APGAR scores of less than four are severely distressed and require immediate resuscitation.

6. ANS—B *PEC—1001*

Presence of fetal meconium at birth indicates the possibility of fetal respiratory distress. Aspiration of meconium can cause severe lung inflammation and pneumonia in the neonate. If you spot meconium during delivery, do not induce respiratory effort until you have removed the meconium from the trachea by suctioning under direct visualization with the laryngoscope. This is a true emergency.

7. ANS—D *PEC—1003*

Normal suctioning of the neonate should be performed by bulb syringe or Delee trap and should last no longer than 10 seconds. Meconium should be suctioned through an endotracheal tube.

8. ANS—A *PEC—1003*

As stated in question one, the first step of the inverted pyramid includes drying and warming the infant; positioning the baby head-down at the level of the vagina; suctioning the mouth and nose; and providing tactile stimulation when necessary.

9. ANS—B *PEC—1007*

An infant's best indicator of stress is the heart rate. If the heart rate is greater than 100 and spontaneous respirations are present, continue assessing the baby. If the heart rate is less than 100, begin positive pressure ventilation immediately. If the heart rate is less than 60 beats per minute, or between 60 and 80 after 30 seconds of positive pressure ventilation and supplemental oxygen, begin chest compressions.

10. ANS—A *PEC—1007*

If the infant presents with cyanosis after performing step one of the inverted pyramid, you should then move to step 2 and administer blow-by oxygen.

11. ANS—B *PEC—1008*

If the heart rate is less than 100 or the infant is still cyanotic after performing step 2, immediately move to step 3 and perform bag-valve mask ventilation.

12. ANS—B *PEC—1008*

If the infant's heart rate is less than 80 after performing steps 1, 2, and 3, move to step 4 and perform chest compressions. Encircle the neonates chest and place both of your fingers on the lower 1/3 of the sternum. Compress the sternum 1/3 to 1/2 of the chest's total height at a rate of at least 100/min.

13. ANS—D *PEC—1008*

The infant's heart rate can be best checked by auscultating the heart at the apex, feeling for pulsation at the umbilical cord, or palpating the brachial pulse.

14. ANS—A *PEC—1008*

When performing bag-valve mask ventilation on the neonate the pop-off valve, if present, should be disengaged. This will prevent underinflation of the infant's lungs.

15.

Figure 33-1

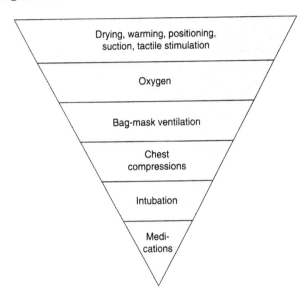

Source: PEC, Figure 33-5.

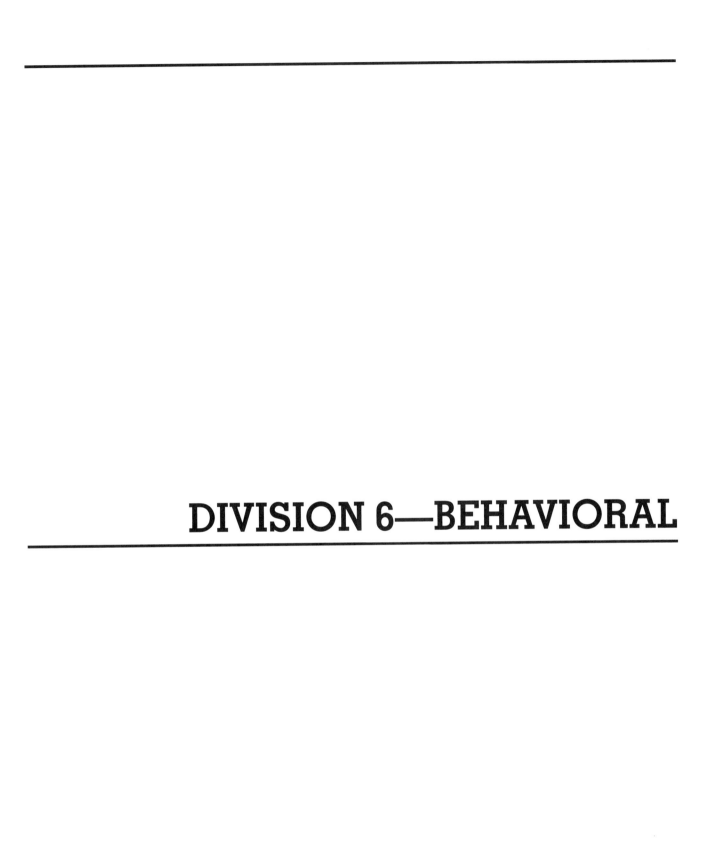

DIVISION 6—BEHAVIORAL

CHAPTER 34

Behavioral and Psychiatric Emergencies

QUESTIONS

1. Which of the following can cause a behavioral emergency?
   A. Underlying psychiatric problem
   B. Substance abuse
   C. Medical illness
   D. All of the above

2. Which of the following interviewing techniques is considered appropriate for the behavioral emergency patient?
   A. Using a formal checklist of questions
   B. Never allowing the patient to lead the interview
   C. Pressing the patient for specific answers
   D. Communicating honesty and firmly

3. During long periods of silence you should
   A. press the patient to keep talking
   B. keep talking yourself
   C. stay calm and relaxed
   D. leave the patient alone

4. If the behavioral emergency patient believes that there are large pink elephants in the room you should
   A. tell him you see them too
   B. understand that they are real for him
   C. tell him there are no pink elephants
   D. tell him he has an obvious psychiatric problem

5. If the distraught patient suddenly begins to cry you should
  A. let them
  B. try to stop them
  C. tell them everything will be all right
  D. start talking

6. Your priority in any behavioral emergency is
  A. your safety
  B. the patient's safety
  C. the underlying reason for the patient's behavioral problem
  D. the patient's life-threatening injuries

7. A mood disorder characterized by feelings of helplessness and hopelessness is
  A. anxiety
  B. depression
  C. mania
  D. schizophrenia

8. Which of the following organic causes can mimic this condition?
  A. Hyperthyroidism
  B. Hypothyroidism
  C. Cushing's disease
  D. Grave's disease

9. Amitriptyline (Elavil), imipramine (Tofranil), and fluoxetine (Prozac) are examples of _____ medications.
  A. antipsychotic
  B. antianxiety
  C. antidepressant
  D. antiparkinson

10. Which of the following is a major suicide risk factor?
  A. Previous attempts
  B. Depression
  C. Widowed spouses
  D. All of the above

11. Which of the following factors increases the risk of the suicide plan?
  A. Well thought out plan
  B. Access to the suicide device
  C. Very lethal method
  D. All of the above

12. Headhache, palpitations, insomnia, and hyperventilation may be signs of
  A. depression
  B. schizophrenia
  C. anxiety
  D. extrapyramidal symptoms

13. Diazepam (Valium), alprazolam (Xanax), and lorazepam (Ativan) are examples of _____ medications.
   A. antipsychotic
   B. antianxiety
   C. antidepressant
   D. antiparkinson

14. A patient with bipolar disorder usually suffers from
   A. frequent hallucinations
   B. wide mood swings
   C. delusional behavior
   D. altered disorganization

15. Lithium (Lithobid) is often prescribed for _____ patients.
   A. schizophrenic
   B. suicidal
   C. organic brain syndrome
   D. manic-depressive

16. The patient who believes he is Jimmy Hoffa and is being chased by mobsters is probably suffering from
   A. manic-depression
   B. paranoid schizophrenia
   C. acute anxiety
   D. none of the above

17. Haloperidol (Haldol) and chlorpromazine (Thorazine) are examples of _____ medications.
   A. antipsychotic
   B. antianxiety
   C. antidepressant
   D. antiparkinson

18. Your patient who exhibits dystonia, dyskinisia, and akathesia may be suffering from
   A. depression
   B. schizophrenia
   C. anxiety
   D. extrapyramidal symptoms

19. Prehospital management of the preceding patient may include
   A. haloperidol (Haldol) IV
   B. diphenhydramine (Benadryl) IV
   C. diazepam (Valium) IV
   D. none of the above

ANSWERS   **1. ANS—D**   *PEC—1014*

Behavioral emergencies can be caused by a number of underlying problems. These include intrapsychic causes (depression, suicide, paranoia, etc.) and organic causes (alcohol, drug abuse, trauma, medical illnesses, dementia, etc.).

2. ANS—D *PEC—1017*

Certain interviewing techniques are appropriate for the behavioral patient. These include communicating self-confidence as well as honesty, firmness, and a reasonable attitude about issues important to the patient and the situation.

3. ANS—C *PEC—1017*

A paramedic should not be afraid of long silent periods during the interview. During this time the paramedic should remain relaxed and attentive.

4. ANS—B *PEC—1017*

Some behavioral patients have delusions. When a patient exhibits delusional behavior, understand that this behavior is reality for this patient.

5. ANS—A *PEC—1017*

Do not disrupt a display of emotion by talking. If a distraught patient suddenly begins to cry, you should simply let them.

6. ANS—A *PEC—1018*

Your top priority in any behavioral emergency is your own personal safety.

7. ANS—B *PEC—1019*

Depression is a common psychiatric disorder. It is characterized by feelings of helplessness and hopelessness.

8. ANS—B *PEC—1019*

Certain organic conditions such as organic brain syndrome, hypothyroidism, or chronic steroid use may mimic depression.

9. ANS—C *PEC—1019*

Amitriptyline (Elavil), imipramine (Tofranil), and fluoxetine (Prozac) are examples of antidepressant medications.

10. ANS—D *PEC—1020*

Some major suicidal risk factors include: previous attempts, history of depression, and widowed spouses.

11. ANS—D *PEC—1020*

Having a well thought out suicidal plan and access to a very lethal suicide device and method all increase the risk of the suicide plan.

12. ANS—C *PEC—1021*

Headache, palpitations, insomnia, and hyperventilation may be signs of an acute anxiety attack. Anxiety is a normal response to stress. However, it can build up to such a point that it overwhelms the patient who then feels helpless and becomes unable to function normally.

13. ANS—B *PEC—1021*

Antianxiety medications such as diazepam (Valium), alprazolam (Xanax), and lorazepam (Ativan), are prescribed for patients who suffer from acute anxiety attacks.

14. ANS—B *PEC—1021*

Bipolar disorder, also called manic-depressive disorder, is a condition characterized by tremendous mood swings from euphoria to debilitating depression.

15. ANS—D *PEC—1021*

Lithium is a drug often prescribed for manic-depressive patients.

16. ANS—B *PEC—1022*

The patient suffering from paranoid-schizophrenia often feels that someone such as the FBI or CIA is after them. Such paranoia often results from the patient's feeling of self importance. Some paranoid-schizophrenics become delusional and believe that they are famous figures such as Jesus Christ or Napoleon.

17. ANS—A *PEC—1022*

Haloperidol (Haldol) and chlorpromazine (Thorazine) are examples of antipsychotic medications.

18. ANS—D *PEC—1023*

Anti-psychotic medications are associated with many side effects. The most common of these are extra-pyramidal symptoms. They include dystonia (impaired muscle tone), dyskinesia (a defect in voluntary movement), and akathesia (inability to sit still).

19. ANS—B *PEC—1023*

Prehospital management of a patient suffering from extra-pyramidal symptoms should include the administration of oxygen, establishment of an IV of normal saline, and the administration of 50 mg of diphenhydramine IV.

12 Lead ECG Monitoring and Interpretation

QUESTIONS

1. Single lead ECG monitoring was principally designed to
   A. diagnose acute myocardial infarction
   B. identify conduction abnormalities
   C. discover physiological problems
   D. detect cardiac dysrhythmias

2. Leads I, II, and III are known as
   A. bipolar limb leads
   B. unipolar limb leads
   C. augmented limb leads
   D. none of the above

3. The remaining leads which read in the frontal plane are the
   A. unipolar limb leads
   B. augmented limb leads
   C. aVr, aVL, aVF
   D. all of the above

4. The precordial leads differ from the limb leads in that
   A. they do not use polarized electrodes
   B. they look at the heart in the horizontal plane
   C. they use the negative electrode as the focal point
   D. they can detect changes in ST segment elevation

5. If the QRS is positive in all three bipolar limb leads, the axis is
   A. deviated to the right
   B. deviated to the left
   C. normal
   D. indeterminate

6. If the QRS is negative in Lead I, positive in Lead III, and variable in Lead II, the axis is
   A. deviated to the right
   B. deviated to the left
   C. normal
   D. indeterminate

7. If the QRS is negative in Leads II and III, the axis is
   A. deviated to the right
   B. deviated to the left
   C. normal
   D. indeterminate

8. Right axis deviation is often associated with
   A. mitral valve disease
   B. high blood pressure
   C. atrial fibrillation
   D. pulmonary hypertension

9. Left axis deviation is often associated with
   A. right heart failure
   B. pulmonary hypertension
   C. asthma
   D. valve disease

10. A depressed ST segment and an inverted T wave are indicative of myocardial
    A. infarction
    B. ischemia
    C. injury
    D. any of the above

11. An elevated ST segment is indicative of myocardial
    A. infarction
    B. ischemia
    C. injury
    D. any of the above

12. A subendocardial infarction is best described as
    A. a partial-thickness injury
    B. a non-Q wave infarction
    C. involving only the deeper myocardial layers
    D. all of the above

13. A Q wave greater than 0.04 seconds in duration is indicative of
    A. myocardial ischemia
    B. normal cardiac function

C. a previous transmural infarction

D. a subendocardial infarction

Match the location of the myocardial ischemia/infarction with the location of ECG changes:

14.	_____ Anterior	**A.**	II, III, aVF, V6
15.	_____ Anteriorlateral	**B.**	V1, V2
16.	_____ Lateral	**C.**	I, V2, V3, V4
17.	_____ High lateral	**D.**	I, aVL, V5, V6.
18.	_____ Inferior	**E.**	V5, V6
19.	_____ Inferolateral	**F.**	I, aVL
20.	_____ True posterior	**G.**	II, III, aVF

ANSWERS

1. ANS—D   *PEC—1031*

Single lead ECG monitoring was designed with a great deal of limitations. It cannot diagnose an MI, conduction abnormalities, or physiological problems. It can only help you detect cardiac dysrhythmias. For this reason, the patient's history remains the most important indicator for suspicion of MI.

2. ANS—A   *PEC—1033*

Leads I, II, and III are known as bipolar limb leads because they basically use two limbs to read the electrical signal in the frontal plane. Lead I reads from right arm to left arm; lead II reads from right arm to left leg; and lead III reads from left arm to left leg.

3. ANS—D   *PEC—1033*

The augmented limb leads, also known as the unipolar limb leads, are aVF, aVL, and aVF. These read using one polarized positive electrode and combined leads that serve as a non-polarized reference point.

4. ANS—B   *PEC—1038*

The precordial leads look at the heart in the horizontal plane. The electrodes are placed across the chest at the fourth and fifth intercostal spaces.

5. ANS—C   *PEC—1041*

If the QRS is not negative in leads I, II, and III, the axis is within normal range.

6. ANS—A   *PEC—1041*

If the QRS is negative in Lead I, positive in Lead III, and variable in Lead II, a right axis deviation exists.

7. ANS—B   *PEC—1041*

If the QRS is negative in Leads II and III, a left axis deviation exists.

8. ANS—D   *PEC—1039*

Right axis deviation is often associated with chronic obstructive pulmonary disease and pulmonary hypertension.

9. ANS—D   *PEC—1039*

Left axis deviation is often associated with high blood pressure and valve disease.

10. ANS—B   *PEC—1044*

A depressed ST segment and an inverted T wave are indicative of myocardial ischemia. The ischemic tissue can depolarize normally but are subject to abnormalities of repolarization.

11. ANS—C   *PEC—1044*

Myocardial injury can result in depolarization abnormalities. The tissue tends to remain depolarized while the surrounding tissues repolarize. This negative charge can be seen as an elevated ST segment on the ECG.

12. ANS—D   *PEC—1044*

A subendocardial infarction is a partial-thickness injury involving only the deeper myocardial layers. It is also known as a non-Q wave infarction.

13. ANS—C   *PEC—1048*

A Q wave greater than 0.04 seconds in duration is indicative of an old transmural infarction. This occurs because of scar tissue that develops in the infarcted area.

14. _____ Anterior	**C.** I, V2, V3, V4
15. _____ Anteriorlateral	**D.** I, aVL, V5, V6.
16. _____ Lateral	**E.** V5, V6
17. _____ High lateral	**F.** I, aVL
18. _____ Inferior	**G.** II, III, aVF
19. _____ Inferolateral	**A.** II, III, aVF, V6
20. _____ True posterior	**B.** V1, V2

Index

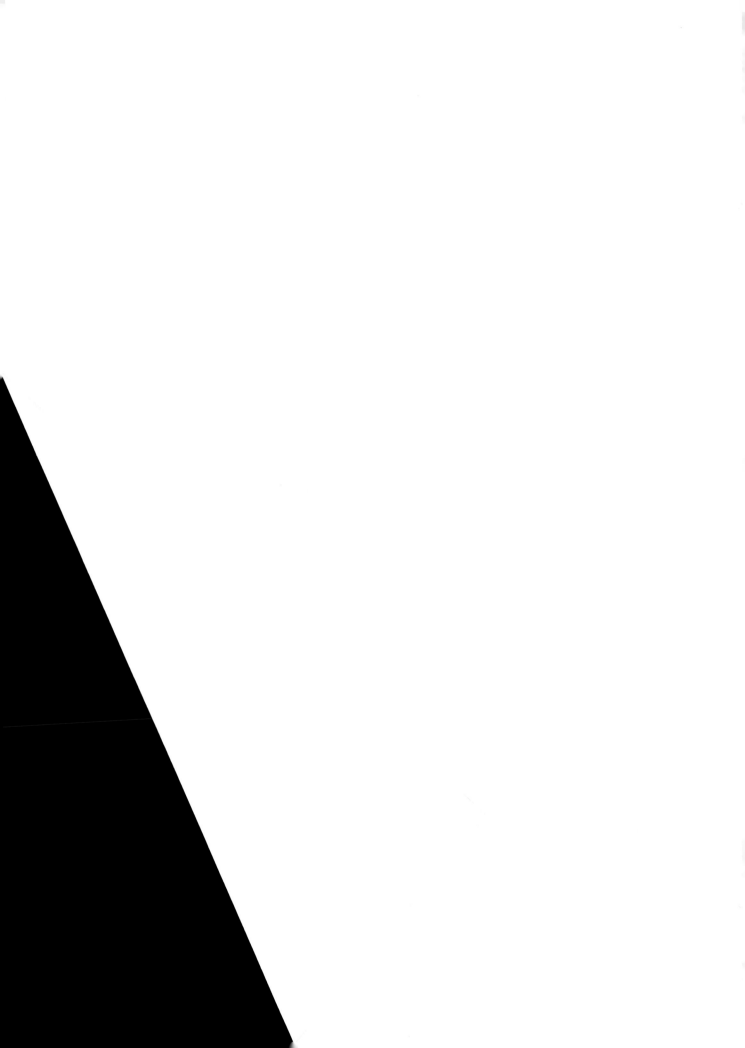